EVIDENCE-BASED MEDICINE & STATISTICS

FOR MEDICAL EXAMS

By **Dr. Marc Barton**
With **Dr. Wolf-Peter Schmidt**

Illustrations by Gareth Baxendale (Gartista™ Original Artworks)

DEDICATION

I dedicate this book to my three wonderful children, Joshua, Emily and Lucy, who amaze and inspire me and make my world a better place to be.

CONTENTS

FOREWORD

Many medical students and I suspect a greater number of doctors look upon statistics with a combination of uncertainty and incomprehension. For some medics, the world of statistics is peopled by a clandestine gang of public health scientists and epidemiologists.

'There are two kinds of statistics: the kind you look up and the kind you make up' wrote Rex Stout, the American author. And yet a good doctor is one who keeps up to date by reading medical journals and publications. It is essential, therefore, to be able to interpret data and critically appraise a research paper; to do so infers that the reader has understood both the 'set up' of the study and the results, and is thus able to formulate his or her own conclusion rather than only accepting the author's findings at face value. Only by adopting such a judicious approach can the reader be able to inform their own clinical practice.

We should not be too ready to dismiss statistics as a dull irrelevance. Far from it. In 1950 Richard Doll and Bradford Hill (later Sir Austin Bradford Hill) showed that smoking was the single most important cause of the rapidly increasing epidemic of lung cancer in the UK. In 1951 they started a prospective study of smoking and mortality in British doctors that Doll continued for 50 years, showing that half of all smokers are eventually killed by their habit and that stopping smoking is remarkably effective.

Evidence-based Medicine and Statistics for Medical Exams is a remarkable book. Its audience will be far wider than that that suggested by the title. Whilst it may be aimed at students sitting undergraduate and postgraduate exams, it will be enormously helpful to practicing doctors and those, too, in allied healthcare professions. It guides the reader through the subject clearly and succinctly, explaining concepts and terms and statistical models.

And all this is achieved with clear text, supportive illustrations, and quizzes at the end of each chapter.

HG Wells said 'statistical thinking will one day be as necessary a qualification for efficient citizenship as the ability to read and write.' This book will go a very long way to help achieve this.

Dr. Michael Barrie
MBBS, MRCGP, DCH, DRCOG, DFFP, DOccMed
GP Principal and author of the highly acclaimed book *The Surgeon's Rhyme*

INTRODUCTION

Statistics and evidence-based medicine are notoriously poorly understood by medical students and doctors. Many students struggle to grasp even the most basic concepts and getting to grips with more the more complex aspects can be truly daunting.

Despite this, these topics have become a vital part of medical practice over recent years. Doctors are now expected to be able to critically appraise scientific papers and journals, and use the information within them to help them to make pragmatic and sensible management decisions with their patients. It is now impossible to stay up-to-date and practice evidenced-based medicine without a solid understanding of medical statistics.

Because of this statistics is now an important part of most medical exams, both at the undergraduate and postgraduate level. This manual is designed to give medical students and doctors a good basic understanding of the principles that they will need to successfully navigate the statistics questions that they are likely to encounter.

Dr Marc Barton
BSc (Hons), MBBS, MRCP, MRCGP, MRCEM, DCH, DRCOG

EVIDENCE-BASED MEDICINE

What is evidence-based medicine?

Evidence-based medicine is the term used to describe the process of systematically reviewing, appraising and using the findings of clinical research to assist with the delivery of optimum clinical care to patients.

The most commonly quoted definition of evidence-based medicine is the one provided by Dr. David Sackett in his 1996 BMJ publication:

'Evidence-based medicine is the conscientious, explicit and judicious use of current best evidence in making decisions about the care of the individual patient. It means integrating individual clinical expertise with the best available external clinical evidence from systematic research.'

The five steps of evidence-based medicine

Evidence-based medicine can be considered to be a 5-step process:

1. **Assess the patient**
    The process of assessing the patient results in the development of a clinical problem.

2. **Ask the question**
    Formulate a well-structured clinical question based upon the clinical problem that has arisen in this case.

3. **Acquire the evidence**
    Search the literature and resources for the best available evidence to answer the clinical question.

4. **Appraise the evidence**

   Review and critically appraise the evidence that you have found assessing it validity, applicability and quality.

5. **Apply your findings**

   Now return to the patient and implement changes based on the evidence that you have discovered. Integrate the evidence with your own clinical expertise but also take into account the preferences of the patient. Monitor this process and self-evaluate your own performance.

The evidence-based medicine triad

It can therefore be seen that the practice of evidence-based medicine can be considered to consist of the following triad:

- Individual clinical expertise
- Best available external clinical evidence
- Patient expectations and values

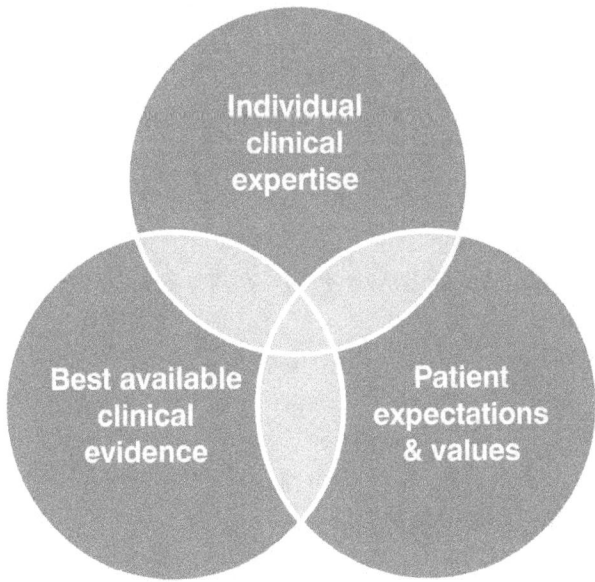

Fig 1. The triad of evidence-based medicine

EVIDENCE-BASED MEDICINE – QUIZ

QUESTIONS

Q1. Which of the following is NOT one of the five-steps of evidence-based medicine?

A. Assessing the patient
B. Formulating a well structured clinical question
C. Commencing a new randomized-controlled trial
D. Critical appraisal of available evidence
E. Implementing changes based on the findings

Q2. Which of the following triads best describes the practice of evidence-based medicine?

A. Individual clinical expertise, budget limitations, guideline production
B. Individual clinical expertise, hospital managers' expectations, initiation of new research
C. Patient expectations and values, budget limitations, hospital managers' expectations
D. Individual clinical expertise, best available external clinical evidence, patient expectations and values
E. Best available external clinical evidence, budget limitations, guideline production

Q3. Which of the following is NOT one of the 5 steps of evidence-based medicine?

A. Assess the patient
B. Ask the question
C. Appraise the evidence
D. Apply your findings
E. Set an appropriate budget

ANSWERS

Q1. C. Commencing a new controlled-controlled trial

Q2. D. Individual clinical expertise, best available external clinical evidence, patient expectations and values

Q3. E. Set an appropriate budget

CLINICAL GOVERNANCE & AUDIT

Clinical governance

Clinical governance refers specifically to the systematic approach of maintaining and improving the quality of patient care within the National Health Service (NHS) in the United Kingdom.

It was defined by Scaly & Donaldson in 1998 as being *'a system through which NHS organizations are accountable for continuously improving the quality of their services and safeguarding high standards of care by creating an environment in which excellence in clinical care will flourish.'*

The domains of clinical governance

Clinical governance is considered to consist of 6 main components, or domains:

1. **Education & training**
    Medicine is a process of lifelong learning and staying up-to-date is of the utmost importance to clinicians and other healthcare professionals. All clinicians working within in the NHS are now expected to undergo a set amount of continuing professional development (CPD) each year.

2. **Clinical audit**
    Clinical audit is *'a quality improvement process that seeks to improve patient care and outcomes through systematic review of care against explicit criteria and the implementation of change.'* (see below)

3. **Clinical effectiveness**

Clinical effectiveness is the process of improving the patients' own personal experience of their healthcare. It involves ensuring that clinical practice is evidence-based and that service delivery is effective.

4. **Research & development**

Best clinical practice is continually changing as a consequence of new evidence from clinical research. It is essential for this research to be evaluated and critically appraised and new practices, guidelines and protocols implemented as a result of the findings.

5. **Openness**

It is very important to learn from mistakes and poor practice. The NHS has developed a culture of openness as part of the clinical governance process. Being open involves acknowledging mistakes, apologizing and explaining what has gone wrong. Investigations should take place so that lessons can be learnt and support should be provided to those involved.

6. **Risk management**

Risk management is the process of identifying, evaluating and correcting potential risks that exist within the organization. These risks can be:

- Risks to patients
- Risks to clinicians and other healthcare professionals
- Risks to the organization itself

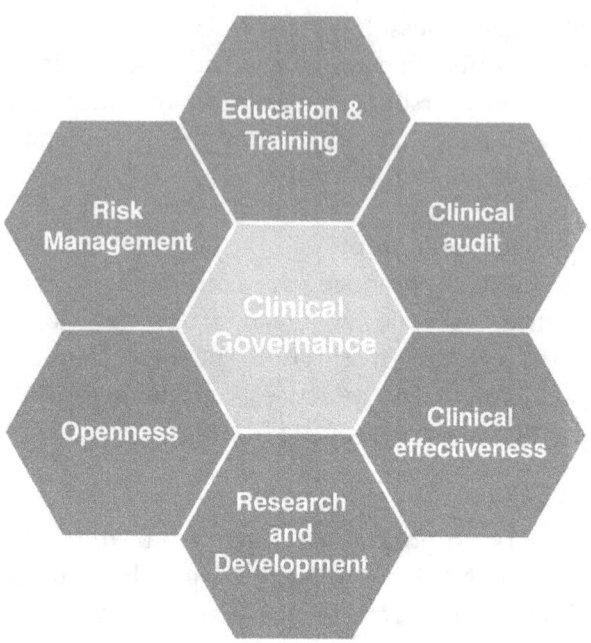

Fig 2. The domains of Clinical Governance from "What is Clinical Governance" by N.Starey

What is clinical audit?

Clinical audit is defined as being '*a quality improvement process that seeks to improve patient care and outcomes through systematic review of care against explicit criteria and the implementation of change.*' It is one component of the NHS clinical governance system and is considered to be a vitally important part of the maintenance and improvement of clinical practice standards.

The audit cycle

The process of clinical audit is a cycle that consists of five set processes as follows:

1. Identification of a problem or an issue
2. Defining the criteria and the setting of standards

3. Observation of practice and data collection
4. Comparison of performance with the criteria and standards
5. Implementation of change

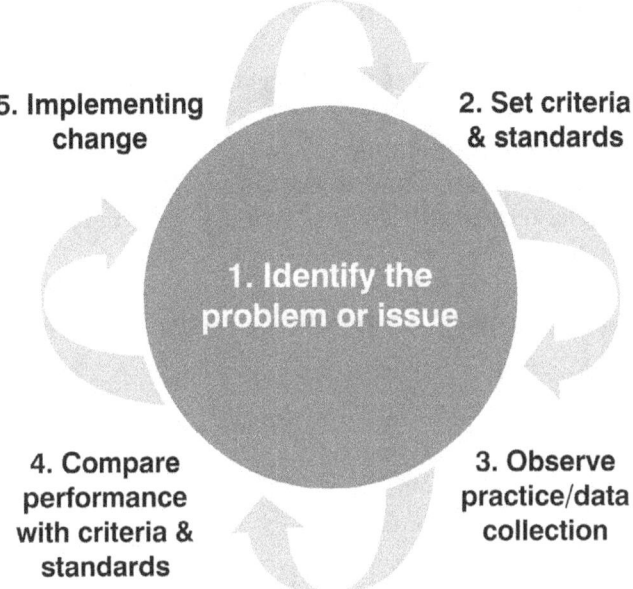

Fig 3. The clinical audit cycle

CLINICAL GOVERNANCE & AUDIT – QUIZ

QUESTIONS

Q1. There are 5 set processes that comprise a clinical audit cycle. Each of these processes are listed below:

1. Observation of practice and data collection
2. Identification of a problem
3. Implementation of change
4. Defining the criteria and the setting of standards
5. Comparison of performance with the criteria and standards

Which is the correct order that these should occur?

A. 1,5,2,4,3
B. 2,4,5,1,3
C. 5,2,4,3,1
D. 2,4,1,5,3
E. 3,4,2,5,1

Q2. Which of the following is NOT one of the 6 domains of clinical governance?

A. Clinical audit
B. Research & development
C. Openness
D. Risk management
E. Government regulation

ANSWERS

Q1. D. 2,4,1,5,3

Q2. E. Government regulation

TYPES OF STUDY

Categories of study design

The type of study design that is chosen depends greatly upon the type of clinical question that is being asked. Broadly speaking there are two different types of medical study:

- Observational studies
- Experimental studies

In observational studies, pre-defined groups are observed to see what happens, or has happened, to them. The different types of observational study consider events or aetiological factors (risk factors) in the past, present or future in an attempt to identify differences between the groups.

Examples of observational studies include:

- Cross-sectional studies
- Cohort studies
- Case-control studies
- Ecological studies

The definition of an experiment is 'a scientific procedure undertaken to make a discovery, test a hypothesis or demonstrate a known fact'. Experimental studies are characterized by introduction of a treatment, procedure or investigation. The results or outcome is then observed and subsequently evaluated.

Cross-sectional studies

A cross-sectional study is a type of observational study that involves collecting data on the presence of disease and risk factors for the disease at the same time in an individual. Individuals are enrolled into the study regardless of disease status (unlike in case control studies). Cross-sectional studies can therefore be used to assess the prevalence of a condition, to answer questions about the cause of a disease, or to assess the results of a medical intervention.

In cross-sectional studies it is often hard to differentiate between cause and effect or establish the sequence of events as risk factors and presence of disease are assessed simultaneously. There is a risk of mixing up cause and effect (reverse causality). For example, when studying the association between diabetes and obesity, it may be unclear whether obesity caused diabetes or diabetes causes the obesity. Cross sectional studies are also not particularly suitable for the study of rare diseases, as huge numbers of individuals may need to be enrolled in order to obtain a sufficient number of cases.

Advantages of cross-sectional studies include:

- Quick to perform
- Can establish association by calculating risk ratios
- Can be used to study multiple outcomes and exposures
- Can be used particularly to study conditions of long duration (e.g. HIV infection or hypertension)

Disadvantages of cross-sectional studies include:

- Moderately expensive to run
- Need large groups
- Sequence of events may remain unclear with a risk of reverse causality
- Conditions of short duration may be hard to catch in a single cross-sectional survey (unless they are very common e.g. influenza-like illnesses)

Cohort studies

A cohort study is a longitudinal, observational study that follows a group of individuals (the cohort) forward in time to monitor the effects of a proposed aetiological factor upon them. In some ways it is the opposite of a case-control study, in which individuals are selected on the basis of whether or not they have a certain disease, and then assessed for the presence or absence of a risk factor under study. In a cohort study, individuals are selected based on the presence or absence of the risk factor (the exposure) under study and then followed up to see whether they develop the disease of interest. As a result, the researcher is able to calculate the incidence risk or the incidence rate of disease in each exposure group and calculate the absolute and relative risk associated with being exposed.

An example of a cohort would be a group of patients that have been exposed to a particular drug. This group could then be followed longitudinally to see if they develop a particular side effect or disease as a consequence of this drug exposure. The comparison group can be the general population from which the cohort was drawn, or alternatively another subgroup of the cohort itself.

Because of the option to select individuals based on their exposure status, cohort studies are good at investigating rare exposures as the study design sets the exposure. A rare outcome is unlikely to appear during the study time and they are therefore poor are detecting rare outcomes, unless the study is very large. Therefore, cohort studies investigating risk factors for cancer or cardiovascular disease often include tens of thousand individuals followed up for 5 to 10 years or even longer.

A cohort study that enrolls individuals at random regardless of their exposure status is called a population based cohort study. This design, in addition to allowing the calculation of the incidence in each exposure group, also allows the calculation of the overall incidence of disease in the total population. This would otherwise be obscured by arbitrarily choosing the number of exposed and unexposed individuals. Cohort studies are practically the only study design that allows the determination of the incidence of a disease.

Being purely observational, the distribution of risk factors in the population is not random, but almost always associated with other factors, which in turn may be associated with the disease of interest. This may lead to confounding and cohort studies are no less subject to confounding than cross-sectional or case control studies.

Advantages of cohort studies include:

- Can assess the sequence of events over time
- Provide information on a wide range of outcomes
- Can be used to study a wide range of exposures
- The risk of selection bias is smaller than in a case control study as risk factors are assessed before a study participant develops disease

Disadvantages of cohort studies include:

- Expensive to run
- Long in duration
- Loss to follow-up can be a significant problem
- Disease outcomes and aetiologies can alter over time

Case-control studies

A case-control study is a type of observational study in which two groups of patients, one with the disease and one without, are compared on the basis of a proposed causative factor that occurred in the past. For example, a researcher may enroll 100 patients with lung cancer treated at one hospital to study risk factors for the disease, by assessing for the presence or absence of these factors in each of them. The researcher chooses a certain number of control individuals (usually between equal numbers and up to 4 times as many) without the disease to assess for the presence or absence of the same risk factors. Crucially, the researcher determines the ratio of diseased and non-diseased individuals in the study and as a consequence disease prevalence or incidence cannot be estimated from case control studies. Cases and controls can be enrolled retrospectively or prospectively, but the assessment of risk factors is usually retrospective.

Case-control studies are suitable to be used when investigating a rare disease or as a preliminary study in cases where little is known about the disease and the proposed aetiological factor. They can look at multiple risk factors (exposures) but can only look at a single outcome.

Case-control studies also allow the assessment of the influence of predictors on outcome via the calculation of an odds ratio. In fact the odds ratio is the only outcome that can be estimated in a case-control study, as prevalence and incidence of the disease will remain unknown.

Bias, and in particular recall and selection bias, are significant problems with case-control studies. An example of recall bias would be cancer patients altering their response to probing questions (e.g. exposure to X-ray related radiation) because they may have thought much more about potential past exposures than healthy individuals. The biggest threat to case-control studies is selection bias. The researcher needs to demonstrate that the controls are from the same source population as the cases. For example, in a hospital-based case control study, the researcher needs to identify controls that would have come to the same hospital had they fallen ill with the same disease. In practice this can be very difficult.

A nested case-control study attempts to combine the advantages of case-control studies (ability to restrict the number of non-diseased individuals in the study) with that of a cohort study (low risk of selection bias as individuals are enrolled before disease develops). Within a large cohort study conducted for some other, more general research objective, newly diagnosed cases of a disease of interest are enrolled, while choosing controls at random from the remaining non diseased population. Risk factors for the disease under study only need to be assessed in these cases and controls and not in the whole cohort population.

Advantages of case-control studies include:

- Relatively inexpensive
- Easy to carry out
- Quick to perform

Disadvantages of case-control studies include:

- Recall bias
- Selection bias

Experimental studies

Experimental studies are characterized by the fact that the study subjects are allocated by the investigator to the different study groups through the use of randomization. Randomization of a sufficiently large number of individuals usually minimizes, if not removes, the potential for confounding as the exposure of interest (usually the treatment) is allocated by chance, independent of other factors associated with disease that study participants may have. Randomization, however, does not eliminate the risk of bias.

Clinical trials are experimental studies and may be:

1. **Un-blinded:**
   these are also known as 'open studies'. Both the patient and the researcher (or treating clinician) are aware of the treatment type

2. **Single-blind:**
   where either the patient or the researcher (or the treating clinician) is not aware which treatment the patient has been randomized to. In these studies it is usually the patient that is unaware of the treatment type.

3. **Double-blind:**

   where neither the patient nor the investigator (or the treating clinician) are aware or which treatment the patient has been randomized to receive.

4. **Triple-blind:**

   a double-blind study in which, in addition, the identities of those enrolled in the study and control groups are also withheld from the statistician who conducts the analysis of the data.

Crossover studies

The crossover design is a modification of the randomized controlled trial in which each patient receives both treatment and placebo in a random order.

Crossover studies are generally only suitable for chronic diseases that are not curable but for which treatment may give short-lived, temporary relief. They are particularly helpful when the outcome is measured by reports of subjective symptoms, such as pain relief from an analgesic, or relief from wheezing in chronic asthma. Outcome is monitored during each period of treatment, and in this way each patient can serve as his own control, which may reduce the number of patients needed to demonstrate an effect.

There is often a 'wash-out' period between tests to remove any carry over effects from the treatment.

Intention-to-treat analysis

Intention-to-treat (ITT) analysis can be used to offset the effects of non-compliance with an intervention. It refers to the inclusion of all study participants in the analysis as part of the group to which they were allocated. They are included regardless of whether or not they completed the study or received the treatment they were allocated.

Intention-to-treat analysis is the only way that the original un-confounded random allocation of a randomized controlled trial can be preserved. It is the only analysis approach where comparability of the two groups is almost guaranteed. This is in contrast to the so-called per-protocol analysis where individuals in the treatment arm who did not comply with the treatment are excluded from the analysis, whilst nobody is excluded from the control arm.

This usually introduces selection bias as individuals with poor compliance may have lower socio-economic status, a lower level of education and an associated higher risk of adverse outcomes. Excluding these individuals from the treatment arm often results in spuriously beneficial treatment effects. Intention-to-treat analysis therefore often signifies a higher quality study methodology.

Intention-to-treat analysis may become problematic if non-compliance with the treatment is very common, for example more than 20% of the trial population. In this case the effect size calculated using the intention-to-treat approach becomes diluted, as many people who did not take the treatment despite being allocated to the treatment group are included in the analysis as if they had taken the treatment. The intention-to-treat analysis does not then reflect the actual treatment effect but instead reflects an average effect in compliers and non-compliers.

Advanced statistical methods, such as the Complier Average Causal Effect (CACE) are sometimes used to deal with this problem. In the CACE approach quite complex statistical models are used to predict the outcome in individuals likely to have been compliant with the treatment had they originally been allocated to the treatment arm. The comparison of this group with the actual compliers in the treatment arm often results in a fairly realistic effect estimate, somewhere between the biased per-protocol analysis and the diluted intention-to-treat analysis.

TYPES OF STUDY – QUIZ

QUESTIONS

Q1. Which of the following statements regarding crossover studies is true?

A. They are a type of observational study
B. Fewer patients are generally needed compared with non-crossover studies
C. They are only suitable for curable diseases
D. No randomization occurs
E. They are not suitable for chronic diseases

Q2. Which of the following is an example of an observational study?

A. Double-blind trial
B. Single-blind trial
C. Crossover study
D. Cohort study
E. Open study

Q3. Which of the following is an example of an experimental study?

A. Crossover study
B. Case-control study
C. Cohort study
D. Cross-sectional study
E. Ecological study

Q4. Which of the following statements about case-control studies is true?

A. They are a type of experimental study
B. They are suitable to be used in the study of rare diseases
C. They are usually more expensive to run than a randomized controlled trial
D. They provide more evidence for causal inference than a randomized controlled trial
E. They are usually longer in duration than prospective cohort studies

Q5. Which of the following statements about cross-sectional studies is true?

A. They are longitudinal in nature
B   They are suitable for the study of rare diseases
C. They can only study a single outcome
D. They can be used to assess the prevalence of a condition
E. They can be used to differentiate between cause and effect

Q6. Which of the following statements about cohort studies is true?

A. They are a type of experimental study
B. They look at groups of patients with the disease being studied
C. They are longitudinal in nature
D. They are the best way to determine the prevalence of a disease
E. They are usually shorter in duration than case-control studies

ANSWERS

Q1. B. Fewer patients are generally needed compared with non-crossover studies

Q2. D. Cohort study

Q3. A. Crossover study

Q4. B. They are suitable to be used in the study of rare diseases

Q5. D. They can be used to assess the prevalence of a condition

Q6. C. They are longitudinal in nature

CONFOUNDING, BIAS & EFFECT MODIFICATION

Confounding factors

A confounding factor is a variable that is associated with both the outcome of interest and the exposure of interest. In this constellation, the exposure of interest appears (spuriously) to be associated with the outcome of interest, while in reality it is the confounding factor (the "third variable") that causally affects the outcome. Importantly, a variable is not considered a confounder if it lies on the causal pathway between the exposure of interest and the outcome.

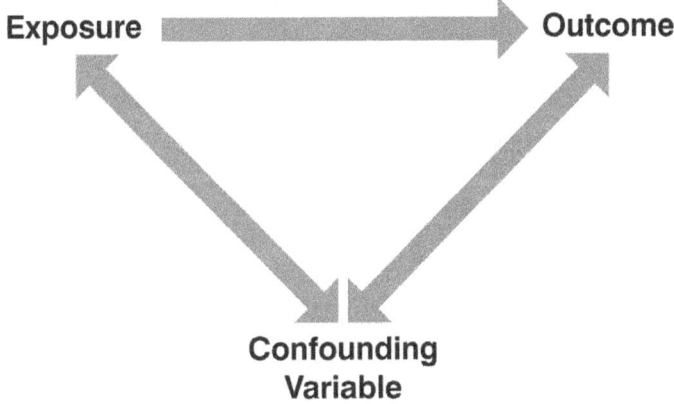

A commonly quoted example of a study that has a confounding variable is one that established a link between coffee consumption and myocardial infarction (MI). Coffee drinkers were indeed found to have an increased risk of suffering a MI. The confounding factor in this case is that coffee drinkers also smoke more significantly and that the increased risk of MI is actually attributable to this.

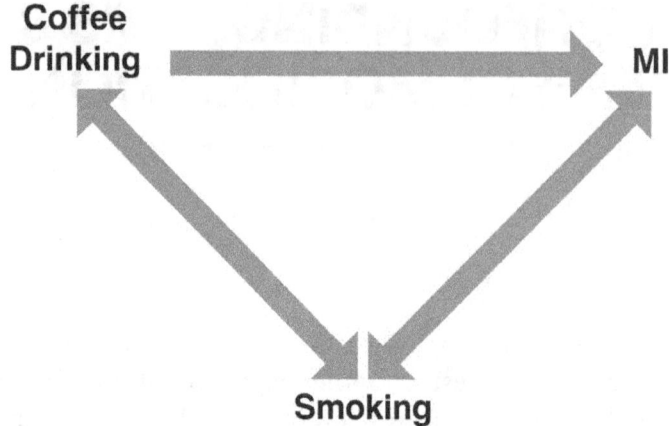

Confounding can result in:

- The observation of a difference between study populations when one does not exit
- The failure to observe a difference between study populations when one actually exists
- The underestimation of an effect
- The overestimation of an effect

Confounding factors need to be accounted for by the researcher. There are two commonly applied ways to do this:

1. **Stratification:**
   In the example of the coffee drinker study, participants are grouped into two groups, smokers and non-smokers. The risk ratio associated with coffee drinking is then calculated within each group separately and then pooled. The resulting pooled risk ratio is then "adjusted (or controlled) for" smoking.

2. **Multivariable regression analysis:**
   This is a more complex approach that uses statistical models (e.g. logistic regression for binary outcomes, linear regression for quantitative outcomes or Cox-regression for survival data) to adjust for confounders. In contrast to stratification, the regression approach allows adjusting (or controlling) for multiple confounders at the same time.

Distinguishing between causal and non-causal association may be difficult. For example, if one were to study the effect of hypertension on the risk of stroke, should one adjust for diabetes, which is may be both causally and non-causally related to hypertension? To help with such decisions, researchers increasingly make use of directed acyclic graphs (DAG) to guide the statistical modeling approach.

Bias

Bias is a systematic error in the way a trial is designed or run resulting in an inaccuracy in the result. While confounding is a problem due to particular characteristics of the study population, bias is a problem due to the study design itself. Confounding can be eliminated by randomization, which balances all potential confounders equally among groups. By contrast, randomization is usually of little help in the avoidance of bias.

There are numerous types of bias that can occur at various stages of the study process. Most forms of bias can be grouped as follows

1. Selection bias
2. Performance bias
3. Measurement bias
4. Publication bias

Selection bias

Selection bias occurs when the groups compared differ systematically in the way participants were enrolled into the study or dropped out from the study. For example, selection bias commonly occurs in case-control studies if controls are selected that come from a different source population than the cases (e.g. they would not have come to that hospital had they fallen ill with the same disease). In a randomized controlled trial comparing a drug (e.g. ACE inhibitor) against placebo, more people in the drug arm may drop out of the study because they experience side effects of the treatment (e.g. cough due to the ACE inhibitor). Dropping out of a study is commonly associated with lower socio-economic status, which in turn is associated with poor health outcomes. Selection bias in this case gives the spurious impression that the drug is effective. Because of side effects, high-risk individuals are more likely to drop out from the active arm than from the control arm. This is sometimes called attrition bias.

Neyman bias (prevalence-incidence bias) is a specific form of selection bias that occurs in case-control studies when the prevalence of a condition does not reflect its incidence. For example, if a disease is characterized by early fatalities and a significant period of time has elapsed between exposure and case selection the 'worst cases' may have already died.

Berkson bias (admission bias) is another example of selection bias that occurs when the hospital admission rate of controls and cases are different from one another because the combination of exposure to risk and occurrence of disease increases the likelihood of being admitted to hospital. This produces a systematically higher exposure rate amongst hospital patients and distorts the odds ratio.

Another example of selection bias is diagnostic purity bias. This occurs when patients with a co-morbidity are excluded from a study. In these circumstances the sample will no longer reflect the true complexity of the population.

Performance bias

Performance bias occurs when systematic differences exist between the care provided to the different intervention groups in the study that is actually part of the treatment of interest. The observed effect of a certain treatment may be spurious. In reality it may be the increased attention given to patients in the treatment arm that improves their outcome.

Measurement bias

Measurement bias occurs when the way that an outcome is assessed produces systematically different results in the two groups compared. Often, it is the knowledge by the patient (the responder) or the researcher (the observer) of the group to which a patient is allocated that leads to measurement bias. Measurement bias is therefore often subdivided into observer and responder bias.

Observer bias occurs when knowledge of treatment allocation causes an 'observer' of the research (i.e. the research team) to fail to properly or impartially measure the outcomes correctly.

Responder bias occurs when knowledge of group allocation changes the behavior of a patient, or the way he responds to questions. A common form of responder bias is recall bias, where participants are aware of their treatment or exposure status and therefore knowingly or unknowingly alter their response to questions asked by the observer. For example, the anxiety experienced by cancer patients may cause them to more acutely remember past episodes of radiation exposure (e.g. X-ray) than control individuals without cancer. Another example is when an intervention aimed at smoking cessation may cause smokers in the intervention arm to lie about their current smoking status for fear of being seen as non-compliant with the intervention. Control individuals who did not receive the smoking cessation intervention may more often correctly report their current smoking status.

The Hawthorne effect, also known as the observer effect, refers to a phenomenon by which people alter or modify their behavior, usually in a positive manner, due to the fact that they are being observed in a research study. The Hawthorne effect, however, only leads to bias if the change in behavior due to being observed differs across the groups compared in a study. Then it is similar to performance bias except that it is not the staff involved in the treatment of patients, but the patients themselves who alter their behavior.

Publication bias

Publication bias occurs when the results of published studies are systematically different from the results of unpublished studies. In these circumstances reviewers are in danger of drawing the wrong conclusion about what the body of research shows. This can potentially have dangerous consequences for patients.

A well-known example of this was the withdrawal of the anti-inflammatory drug Vioxx (rofecoxib) due to safety concerns by its producer Merck. Media reports accused Merck of having prevented the publication of studies that indicated a high prevalence of cardiovascular events in patients taking Vioxx long-term. If this was true and this data had been published a different conclusion about the safety of Vioxx may have been drawn at an earlier stage.

Effect modification

Effect modification (interaction) occurs if the effect of a risk factor on an outcome measure differs between different levels of a third variable (for example gender, ethnicity or smoking status). Smoking status is a common effect modifier. A classic, but somewhat controversial, example concerns the finding that asbestos exposure may disproportionally increase the risk of lung cancer in those exposed to asbestos that are also smokers. Asbestos exposure alone increases the risk of lung cancer 3 fold, which is a risk ratio of 3. Smoking alone is thought to increase the risk of lung cancer 10 fold (risk ratio of 10). In the absence of effect modification, we would expect that those exposed to both asbestos and smoking to have a 30 times higher risk (3 x 10) of lung cancer than those who don't smoke and are not exposed to asbestos. However, some (but not all studies) have suggested that the risk associated with the combined exposure (smoking and asbestos) compared to those exposed to neither is much higher than 30, and may be as high as 60. The effects of smoking and asbestos exposure have combined to have a multiplicative effect. Asbestos and smoking are then said to be *interacting*, because the combined effect is greater than one would expect.

It should be noted that it would still be called an effect modification or interaction if the combined effect were smaller than expected, for example if the risk of lung cancer due to asbestos exposure were smaller in smokers than in non-smokers.

In rare cases, effect modification can even lead to a factor being a risk factor in some people (e.g. women), but a protective factor in others (e.g. men). On average, these two effects would cancel out and we would see no effect in the total population.

Unlike confounding, effect modification is a biological phenomenon in which the exposure has a different impact in different circumstances, which may be of scientific interest. Often, however, one will find evidence for differences in effects among various subgroups by chance alone. Unless there is a good biological reason to suspect effect modification, differences in effects among groups are likely to be due to chance and should not be given too much importance until a further study has confirmed the finding.

CONFOUNDING, BIAS & EFFECT MODIFICATION – QUIZ

QUESTIONS

Q1. Which type of bias occurs when the prevalence of a condition does not reflect its incidence?

A. Diagnostic purity bias
B. Berkson bias
C. Historical control bias
D. Neyman bias
E. Recall bias

Q2. Which type of bias can occur when patients with a co-morbidity are excluded from a study?

A. Berkson bias
B. Neyman bias
C. Diagnostic purity bias
D. Membership bias
E. Historical control bias

Q3. Which type of bias occurs when the number of patients dropping out of the study differs significantly between the groups being investigated?

A. Historical control bias
B. Performance bias
C. Recall bias
D. Response bias
E. Attrition bias

Q4. Which type of bias occurs when the act of observing people alters the way in which they behave?

A. Hawthorne effect
B. Neyman bias
C. Diagnostic purity bias
D. Performance bias
E. Berkson bias

Q5. Which of the following best describes a confounding factor?

A. Prior knowledge of clinical data influencing the outcome of the resulting diagnostic process
B. A variable that has not been controlled or eliminated by the researcher
C. The number of patients dropping out of a study differing significantly between the groups being investigated
D. A systematic error in the way a trial is designed or run resulting in an inaccuracy in the result
E. Subjects answering in a way they think the researcher will want them to

ANSWERS

Q1. D. Neyman bias

Q2. C. Diagnostic purity bias

Q3. E. Attrition bias

Q4. I. Hawthorne effect

Q5. B. A variable that has not been controlled or eliminated by the researcher

RANDOMIZATION

Randomization

In experimental studies there are usually many factors acting as confounders that are not measured, or not measured with sufficient accuracy. These are called unknown confounders. The only way to deal with unknown confounders is randomization.

Randomization is the process by which an individual has an equal chance of entering any group within a study. It serves to reduce confounding by distributing characteristics of patients that may influence outcomes randomly between the groups. There are a number of potential methods of randomization:

1. **Simple randomization:**
    Simple randomization can be thought of as being akin to tossing a coin. A numbered list is created linking set numbers of patients to a particular group in sequence. The investigators can use random number tables, random functions on calculators or statistical software to generate the list.

2. **Block randomization:**
    Block randomization occurs when subjects are placed into 'blocks' which, when filled, are divided equally into the two different arms of the study. This ensures that there are equal numbers of subjects in each arm. The main disadvantage of block randomization is that the allocation of participants can be predicted by researchers and this may result in selection bias. This is why many trials employ varying block sizes (often between 4 and 8) so that investigators cannot predict allocation on the basis of previous patients.

3. **Stratified randomization:**
    Stratified randomization can be used when a potential confounding factor is known. For example, if it is already

known that smoking status and gender highly affect the study outcome, it may be worthwhile stratifying the study population by these two factors; this results in 4 groups (male/smoker, female/smoker, male/non-smoker, female/non-smoker). Randomization is then carried out within each subgroup separately. This guarantees that these known confounders are balanced across trial arms.

4. **Cluster randomization:**

Cluster randomization occurs when groups of subjects, as opposed to individual subjects, are randomized. An example would be when patients are randomized according to the hospital that they present to. The hospital would therefore become the unit of randomization rather than the individual. The main problem with cluster randomization is that it reduces the statistical power to detect an effect. In other words, more patients are needed in a cluster randomized trial compared to an individual randomized trial. This is because the ability of a randomized controlled trial to detect a certain effect size with sufficient accuracy (study power) largely depends on how often random allocation is done, i.e. how often "the coin is tossed". In an individual randomized trial, the coin is tossed once for every individual. In a cluster randomized trial the coin is tossed once for every group of patients. The factor by which the number of patients in a trial needs to be increased due to cluster randomization as opposed to individual randomization is called the 'Design Effect'.

5. **Minimization:**

Minimization is an example of an 'adaptive randomization' method. With minimization a running total is kept of all the levels of the prognostic factors of interest. The first patient in the trial is randomly allocated but all subsequent patients are randomized using a randomization weighted towards which assignment would reduce, or minimize, any imbalance. Minimization is useful when multiple factors need to be distributed evenly between the study groups. It is also a good way of ensuring that smaller studies have similar arms.

Allocation concealment

The randomization process is dependant upon effective allocation concealment. This process ensures that both clinicians and participants unaware of the treatment being allocated prior to enrollment in the study. Without it, even well thought out randomization processes can be subverted.

RANDOMIZATION – QUIZ

QUESTIONS

Q1. Which type of randomization occurs when groups of subjects, as opposed to individual subjects, are randomized?

A. Fixed randomization
B. Adaptive randomization
C. Simple randomization
D. Block randomization
E. Cluster randomization

Q2. Which type of randomization can be thought of as being akin to tossing a coin?

A. Fixed randomization
B. Simple randomization
C. Block randomization
D. luster randomization
E. Minimization

Q3. Which type of randomization occurs when a potential confounding factor is known about and separate randomization lists are generated to reduce the effects of this confounding factor?

A. Adaptive randomization
B. Simple randomization
C. Block randomization
D. Cluster randomization
E. Stratified randomization

Q4. Which type of bias can potentially occur due to block randomization?

A. Performance bias
B. Attrition bias
C. Selection bias
D. Diagnostic purity bias
E. Membership bias

ANSWERS

Q1. E. Cluster randomization

Q2. B. Simple randomization

Q3. E. Stratified randomization

Q4. C. Selection bias

END-POINTS & VALIDITY

End-points

An end-point is an outcome measure or event that can be measured to determine whether the intervention being studied is beneficial or not. End-points allow a decision to be made about whether the null hypothesis of that clinical trial can be accepted or rejected. The null hypothesis states that there is no statistically significant difference between two treatments being compared with respect to the endpoint measure chosen.

The end-point of a clinical trial is generally included in the study objectives. An endpoint (or outcome measure) can broadly be categorized as objective (e.g. based on a biomarker, imaging or the diagnosis based on defined criteria by a clinician unaware of treatment allocation) or subjective (e.g. self-report of symptoms such as pain or mood).

Primary vs. secondary end-points

The primary end-point of a study is the main point of interest of the study in question. An example would be to ascertain whether or not a new drug is better at preventing mortality from a clinical condition than older standard therapy.

Secondary end-points are other characteristics that are measured in the study participants that help to answer other relevant questions about the same clinical trial. An example would be whether the same drug mentioned above was cost effective or affected disease measures other than mortality. Many trials with mortality as primary endpoint use non-fatal outcomes (e.g. non-fatal stroke or myocardial infarction) as secondary outcomes with the objective of further exploring the effect of a drug.

Often trials fail to show an effect of a treatment on the primary endpoint while an effect was found for a secondary outcome. In these circumstances it would be inappropriate to conclude that the treatment is effective. Based on a secondary outcome all that can be done is to develop a new hypothesis and perform a further trial to confirm the effect.

Types of end-point

There are, broadly speaking, three main types of study end-point:

1. **Clinical end-points**

    A clinical end-point is a measurement of a direct clinical outcome. Examples of this would include mortality, morbidity, survival, improvements in quality of life or relief of symptoms.

2. **Surrogate end-points**

    A surrogate end-point is a measurement that may correlate with a clinical end-point but is not guaranteed to do so. An example of a surrogate end-point would be the measuring of gastric pH instead of the actual clinical end-point, which would be upper gastrointestinal bleeding.

3. **Composite end-points**

    Composite end-points combine a number of different measurements into a single composite end-point. These sorts of end-point are useful when any single event occurs too infrequently to be used as an end-point on its own. For example, many trials on cardiovascular drug treatments use end-point definitions such as "major cardiovascular event" rather than myocardial infarction. This may help to improve the power of a study.

Validity

Validity is a means of measuring the end-points chosen by a study. It is the extent to which a conclusion, or measurement, is well founded and corresponds accurately to the real world. Validity can be internal or external.

The internal validity of a study is the extent to which the methodology permits a conclusion about causal relationships to be made. It looks at whether the study methodology and design was of a suitable quality to avoid confounding. The less chance for confounding in the study, the higher its internal validity is.

The external validity is the extent to which the results of a study can be extrapolated to other situations and to other people. It is a measure of how the study findings apply to the wider population.

END-POINTS & VALIDITY - QUIZ

QUESTIONS

Q1. Which statistical measure is the main point of interest of a study?

A. Tertiary end-point
B. Surrogate end-point
C. Primary end-point
D. Secondary end-point
E. Composite end-point

Q2. Which type of end-point combines a number of different measurements into a single end-point?

A. Tertiary end-point
B. Surrogate end-point
C. Primary end-point
D. Secondary end-point
E. Composite end-point

Q3. Which type of end-point is mortality and morbidity an example of?

A. Clinical end-point
B. Surrogate end-point
C. Primary end-point
D. Secondary end-point
E. Composite end-point

ANSWERS

Q1. C. Primary end-point

Q2. E. Composite end-point

Q3. A. Clinical end-point

PHASES OF CLINICAL RESEARCH

Bringing new drugs onto the market

The process of bringing new drugs (or other health interventions) onto the market is long and arduous and in some cases can take years, or even decades. Developing any new drug begins by developing an understanding of the disease or condition that it is intended to treat.

Basic scientific research provides ideas about potential strategies to target the specific etiology of the condition. Biological targets are identified and drugs are formulated to act on these targets.

The research process starts in the 'pre-clinical phase' with studies at a cellular level and eventually progresses to animal models to determine whether the target is influenced by the drug.

Once the researchers have completed the vigorous pre-clinical screening process they can apply for a clinical trial authorization to allow for the investigational drug to be tested on human volunteers in clinical trials.

Clinical drug trials

A clinical drug trial is a study that is carefully designed to assess the benefits and risks of a specific investigational drug. They usually comprise the following stages, or phases:

Phase 1:
Phase 1 trials are usually small trials that recruit only a small number of healthy volunteers (usually in the region of 20-100 participants). These trials usually last several months. The main

purpose of phase 1 is to gather information on dosing, timing and safety of new drug. There is approximately a 70% success rate and progression to phase 2.

Phase 2:

Phase 2 trials are generally slightly larger than phase 1 (usually in the region of 100-300 participants) and they last longer (up to 2 years). In this phase the drug is tested on patients and the primary goal is to test the safety and effectiveness of the new drug. There is approximately a 33% success rate and progression to Phase 3. It should be noted that some trials cover Phase 2 and 3 together.

Phase 3:

Phase 3 trials usually have several thousand participants depending on the expected size of the effect and the incidence of the study outcome (usually a disease or condition). They evaluate the effectiveness of the new drug compared with existing drugs or placebo and are generally randomized controlled trials. They usually last between 1 and 4 years and have approximately a 25% success rate.

Phase 4:

Phase 4 usually takes the form of post marketing surveillance (see below) and is designed to further track long-term side effects and benefits. They usually have a high success rate (70-90%).

Post-marketing surveillance

Post-marketing surveillance (PMS) is the practice of monitoring the safety of a drug within the patient population after it has been released. Although the drug will have been subjected to numerous clinical trials prior to release, PMS forms an important part of the ongoing assessment of these drugs, because even large phase 3 trials are too small to detect serious side effects unless these are common. The regulatory body responsible for PMS varies from country to country.

In the UK the Medicines and Healthcare products Regulatory Agency (MHRA) and the Commission on Human Medicines (CHM) jointly operates the Yellow Card Scheme, which is aimed at identifying and mitigating Adverse Drug Reactions (ADRs).

In the United States PMS is performed by the Food and Drug Administration (FDA), which operates a system called MedWatch, to which both doctors and patients can voluntarily report ADRs.

In Canada PMS is performed by Health Canada, which has a division responsible for it called Marketed Health Products Directorate (MHPD).

PHASES OF CLINICAL RESEARCH – QUIZ

QUESTIONS

Q1. Which of the following is true regarding Phase 1 drug trials?

A. There are usually several thousand participants
B. They usually last several years
C. They gather information about long-term side effects
D. About 25% progress to Phase 2 trials
E. They gather information about drug dosing

Q2. Which of the following is true regarding Phase 2 drug trials?

A. They gather information about timing of new drugs
B. They study safety and effectiveness of new drugs
C. Most progress to Phase 3 trials
D. They are never combined with Phase 3 trials
E. They are usually several thousand participants

Q3. Which of the following is true regarding Phase 3 drug trials?

A. They gather information about timing of new drugs
B. They study safety and effectiveness of new drugs
C. They usually take the form of a cohort study
D. They evaluate the effectiveness of new drugs compared with existing drugs
E. They have a 90% success rate

Q4. Which of the following is true regarding Phase 4 drug trials?

A. They gather information about dosing of new drugs
B. They study the effectiveness of new drugs
C. They are generally short in duration
D. They have a low success rate
E. They are designed to track long-term side effects of new drugs

Q5. Which of the following is the main advantage of post-marketing surveillance (PMS) of a newly released drug?

A. To assess the cost effectiveness of the drug
B. To assess the safe dose range of drug
C. To assess for Type A drug reactions
D. To assess for patient satisfaction
E. To assess the safety of the drug in the patient population

ANSWERS

Q1. E. They gather information about drug dosing

Q2. B. They study safety and effectiveness of new drugs

Q3. D. They evaluate the effectiveness of new drugs compared with existing drugs

Q4. E. They are designed to track long-term side effects of new drugs

Q5. E. To assess the safety of the drug in the patient population

META-ANALYSIS &
SYSTEMATIC REVIEW

What is meta-analysis?

Meta-analysis is a statistical procedure that integrates the results of multiple independent studies with common features with the goal of estimating the true common effect across these individual trials. By combining studies, a meta-analysis increases the sample size and therefore the power to study the effects of interest. It is useful when individual studies are too small to give reliable answers alone. It has, however, been shown that even large trials on the same treatment may produce conflicting results, which may be due to chance or due to subtle differences in the design of each trial. By conducting subgroup analyses of groups of trials, meta-analyses also allow the investigation of why such differences between studies may have occurred. Meta-analyses are also often used to determine if new studies are needed to further investigate a treatment.

Meta-analysis usually involves the creation of a forest plot showing the effect sizes of all included studies in one graph, along with a marker of the combined effect. The combined effect is essentially an average of the treatment effects identified by the individual studies, with more weight being given to larger studies.

To avoid bias, both positive and negative studies should be included. Research has proven that studies with a positive result are more likely to be published than those with a negative result. This is referred to as 'publication bias' and proper selection of studies for meta-analysis can help to overcome this. In order to avoid bias, unpublished but properly conducted studies should also be included. In many cases this may mean inclusion of studies published in the non-English literature. Many examples exist where the acquisition of previously unpublished data substantially alters the assumed benefit of a drug, often towards no effect or even a detrimental effect. An example of this is the use of selective serotonin receptor inhibitors for the treatment of depression in adolescents. Any meta-analysis therefore needs to follow a strict protocol of identifying studies, exclusion and inclusion criteria and listing strengths and weaknesses of each individual study.

There is a debate in evidence-based medicine as to what extent heterogeneous trials of obviously different methodology should be pooled using meta-analysis. Strictly speaking studies should only be pooled if the treatment under investigation is similar in all the included studies, and differences in the effect size among studies can be assumed to have occurred by chance only. Since most meta-analyses of drug treatment include trials where different dosages have been used this assumption is often violated. Nevertheless, these meta-analyses provide indispensable information for clinicians. A different form of meta-analysis, called random effects meta-analysis has been suggested as a way to deal with heterogeneity among studies. This approach however, has a number of theoretical and practical limitations and cannot therefore generally be recommended.

In summary the principal advantages of meta-analysis are as follows:

- Allows the integration and summary of results from individual studies
- Allows analysis of differences in results from individual studies
- Increases precision in estimating effects
- Can overcome small sample sizes

Systematic review

A systematic review is the first step in a meta-analysis and attempts to review systematically all of the pertinent articles relating to a particular research question. A systematic review is very similar to a meta-analysis, the main difference being that no pooled effect is estimated. It is customary in systematic reviews to present a forest plot as in meta-analysis, but without showing the pooled effect (which would in fact make it a meta-analysis).

The most common reasons for only doing a systematic review without a subsequent meta-analysis are:

1. The literature search failed to identify more than one study, or;
2. The studies identified in the literature search were of substantially different methodology precluding the use of meta-analysis.

Systematic reviews of high-quality randomized-controlled trials are now considered to be a vital part of evidence-based medicine. An understanding of systematic reviews and how to implement them in medical practice is now an obligatory part of modern medical practice.

The Cochrane Collaboration

The Cochrane Collaboration is an independent organization that was formed to organize medical research information in a systematic way. This group conducts systematic reviews of randomized-controlled trials focused on health-care interventions, which are published in The Cochrane Library.

The group consists of volunteers, which currently number in excess of 30,000 and are spread across over 120 countries. Their aim is to gather and summarize the best health care evidence from research to enable doctors, nurses and patients make informed choices about treatment.

Cochrane reviews are conducted under a standardized and strictly supervised process of identifying eligible studies, determining the quality of each study and provide a summary of the results with a statement regarding the need for further studies. Study results are ideally summarized in the form of meta-analysis where applicable.

META-ANALYSIS & SYSTEMATIC REVIEW – QUIZ

QUESTIONS

Q1. Which of the following statements regarding meta-analysis of randomized controlled trials is true?

A. Unpublished studies should be excluded
B. They examine variability between studies
C. Only positive studies should be included
D. They should include only large studies
E. They should only include peer-reviewed studies

Q2. Which of the following is NOT an advantage of meta-analyses?

A. They eliminate the need for further studies
B. They can increase the power to study the effects of interest
C. They increase precision in estimating effects
D. They increase precision in estimating effects
E. They can help to overcome 'publication bias'

ANSWERS

Q1. B. They examine variability between studies

Q2. A. They eliminate the need for further studies

PLOTS

Plots in medical statistics

A plot is a graphical method of representing a data set. There are a variety of different types of plots, or graphs, used in studies and a basic understanding of these different plots is essential when attempting to critically appraise the data findings.

Stem and leaf plots

Stem and leaf plots are a very simple method for demonstrating the frequency with which certain classes of values occur. The plot breaks each value of a quantitative data set into two pieces, a stem, typically for the highest place value, and a leaf for the other place values. It provides a way to list all data values in a compact form.

stem	leaf
9	0 4
8	3 4 5 7 9
7	0 2 2 9
6	5 8 9
5	3

Fig 4. A very simple stem and leaf plot

Histograms

A histogram is a graphical representation of the distribution of numerical data. Histograms are particularly useful when there are a large number of observations. Data is displayed using bars of different heights. These bars are created by dividing the entire range of values into a series of intervals, called class intervals. The number of values falling into each interval is then counted to obtain the class frequencies. The height of each bar corresponds to its class frequency.

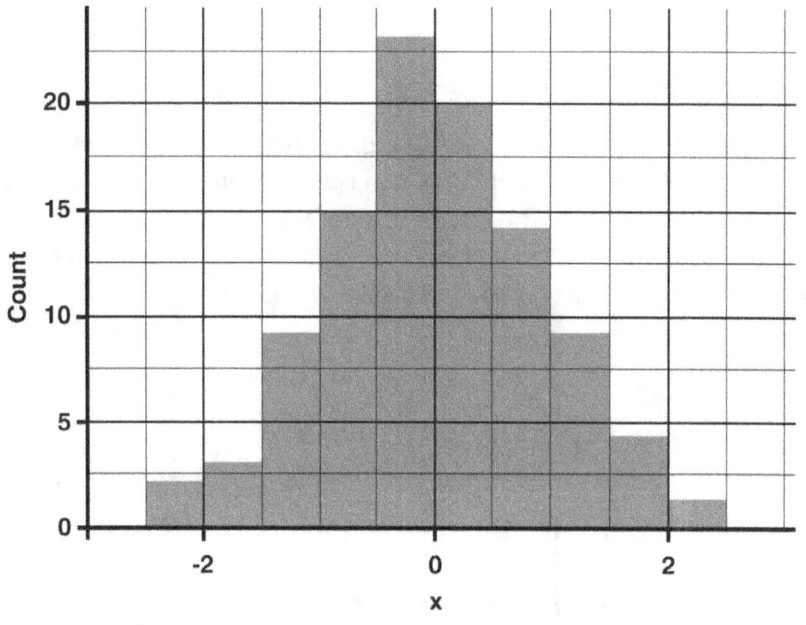

Fig 5. Histogram

Scatterplots

A scatterplot consists of an X axis (the horizontal axis), a Y axis (the vertical axis), and a series of dots. Each dot on the scatterplot represents one observation from a data set. The position of the dot on the scatterplot represents its X and Y values.

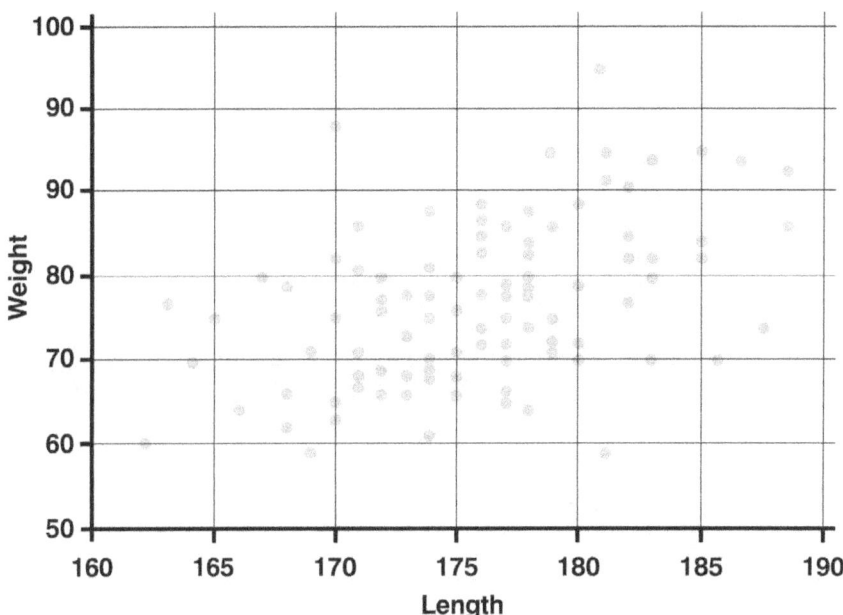

Fig 6. Scatterplot

A scatter plot is used to plot possible related variables graphically. For example, as above, there is a positive correlation between increasing length and weight in the subjects measured. A line of 'best fit' can be drawn to study this correlation.

Pareto diagram

A Pareto diagram (also called a Pareto chart) is a type of chart that contains both a bar graph and a line graph. Each bar represents a category or set of qualitative data. The bars are arranged in order of frequency, so that more important categories are emphasized. The cumulative total is represented by the line graph.

The main purpose of a Pareto diagram is to highlight the most important data set among a set of different factors.

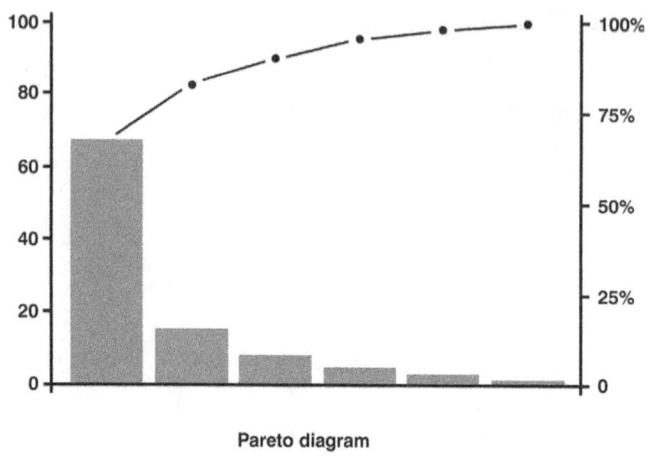

Pareto diagram

Fig 7. Example of a Pareto diagram

Forest plots

A forest plot graphically displays the relative strength of multiple studies that are trying to answer the same question. Forest plots are used in systematic reviews and meta-analysis as a graphical means of illustrating the relative strength of treatment effects in multiple individual studies addressing the same question.

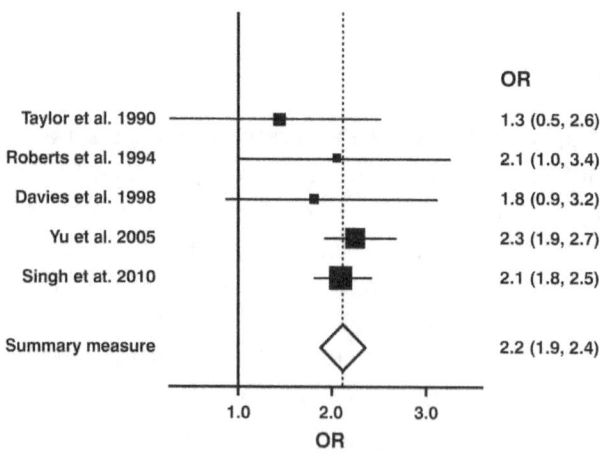

Fig 8. Forest plot

The X column usually lists the names of the studies and the Y column looks at the measure of effect of each of these studies. The area of the squares is proportional to the number of events in each study. The length of the horizontal lines emerging from the squares represents the confidence interval. The diamond at the bottom of the plot shows the average effect size of the studies combined, this effect size is called meta-analysis. Systematic reviews where meta-analysis is not possible (usually because individual studies are too different in methodology to be comparable) often use a forest plot that omits the summary measure (the diamond).

Funnel plots

Funnel plots are a graphical means of checking for publication bias in meta-analyses and systematic reviews. The basic assumption is that trials showing no effect are less likely to be published if they are small than if they are large. Researchers conducting a large trial (which requires a lot of effort and funding) usually have an interest to publish the trial results even if negative. Furthermore, the running of a large trial is usually widely known in the field and difficult to hide. By contrast, it has been shown that small trials with a negative result more often remain unpublished, possibly because of a lack of interest or because the researcher (who may have links with the drug company funding the trial) may want to hide the negative result from the public. Evidence for publication bias can be assumed if smaller trials show more positive effects than larger trials (because small studies with a negative effects are more likely to remain unpublished).

The vertical axis of a funnel plot is a measurement of the precision of the estimated treatment effect (which is also an approximate measure of the size of the trial). The horizontal axis measures the treatment effect. The point estimate from each study is then plotted onto the graph and a vertical line inserted where the pooled estimate from the meta-analysis will lie. If the dots denoting the individual studies roughly form a symmetrical triangle, then publication bias is probably absent. If there is asymmetry, then publication bias can be suspected.

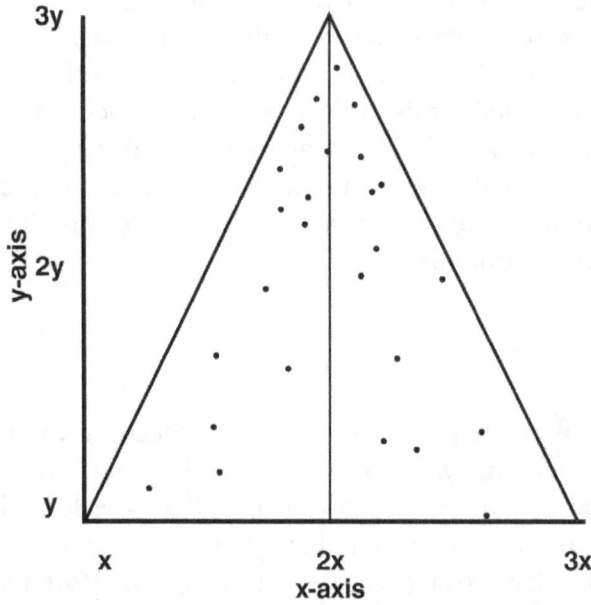

Fig 9. Funnel plot

Box and whiskers plots

A box plot is a means of graphically showing numerical data through its quartiles. The lines extending vertically are known as whiskers and indicate the variability outside the upper and lower quartiles. Individual points outside the whiskers are outliers.

Box plots are non-parametric. The spacing between different parts of the box indicates the amount of spread and the degree of skew in the data collected.

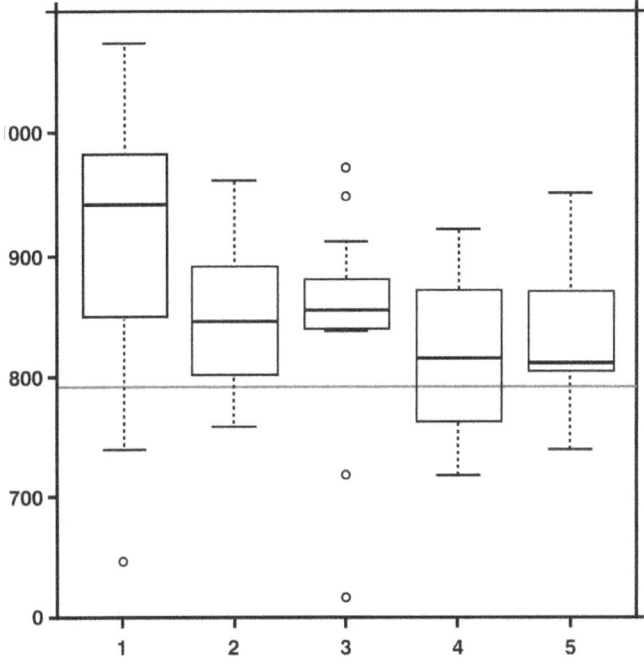

Fig 10. Box and whiskers plot

Box and whisker plots are constructed as follows:

- 75% of the values lie below the upper quartile
- 25% of the values lie below the lower quartile
- The box represents 50% of the data
- The box is divided by the median
- Outliers may be plotted as individual points

L'abbe plot

L'Abbe plots are commonly used to display data visually in a meta-analysis of clinical trials that compare treatments against control intervention or placebos. They are essentially scatter-plots of results of individual studies with the treatment group results on the vertical axis and the control group results on the horizontal axis.

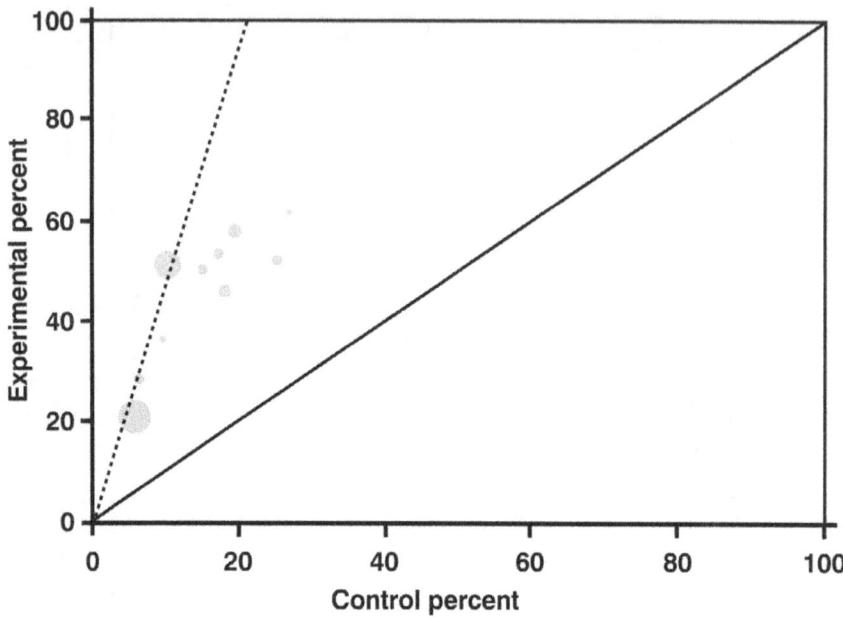

Fig 11. L'abbe plot

Trials in which experimental treatment is better than control are displayed in the upper left hand side of the plot. Trials in which control or placebo are better than the experimental treatment are displayed on the lower right of the plot. The size of the trial is reflected by the size of the circle used.

Cates plot

Cates plots have been used since 1999 as a means of providing visual aid when communicating the risks and benefits of treatments to patients. It consists of green 'smiley faces', that represent good outcomes, and red 'sad faces' that represent bad outcomes.

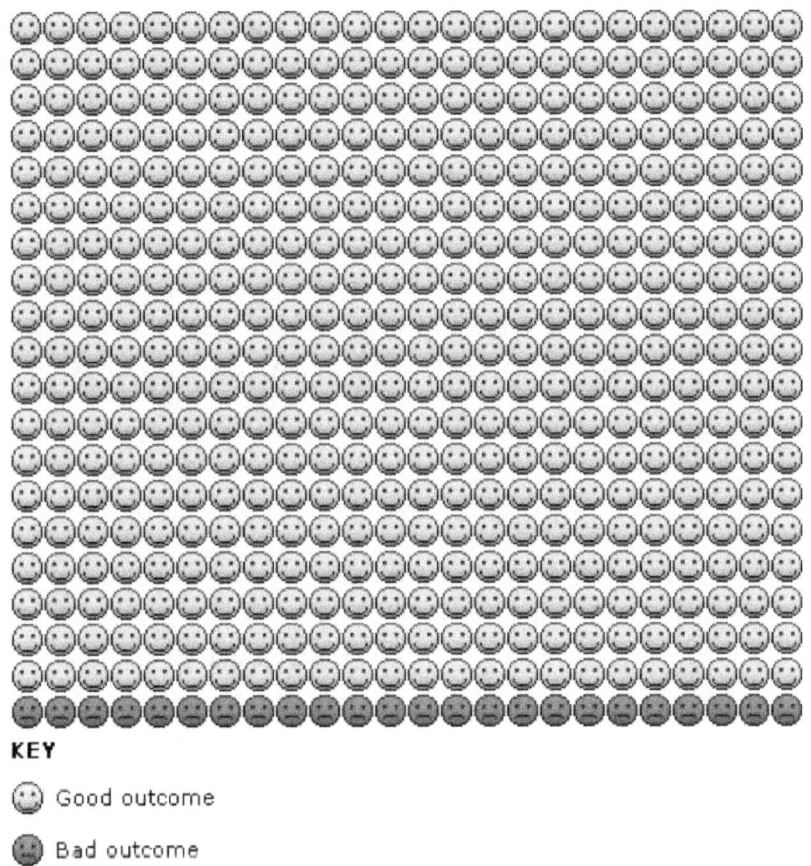

KEY

😊 Good outcome

😞 Bad outcome

Fig 12. Cates plot

Cates plots are widely used in the QRISK® toolkits that are available online and are useful ways of communicating risk of certain disease to patients.

Kaplan-Meier plots

Kaplan-Meier plots provide a useful means of comparing survival times amongst patients receiving different treatments or management protocols. Collected survival data is presented in the form of a survival curve, which is plotted by calculating the proportion of patients who remain alive in the study each time an event occurs. The plot that is created takes the form of a series of declining horizontal steps. Time is plotted on the X axis and the proportion of people that have survived at each time point is plotted on the Y axis.

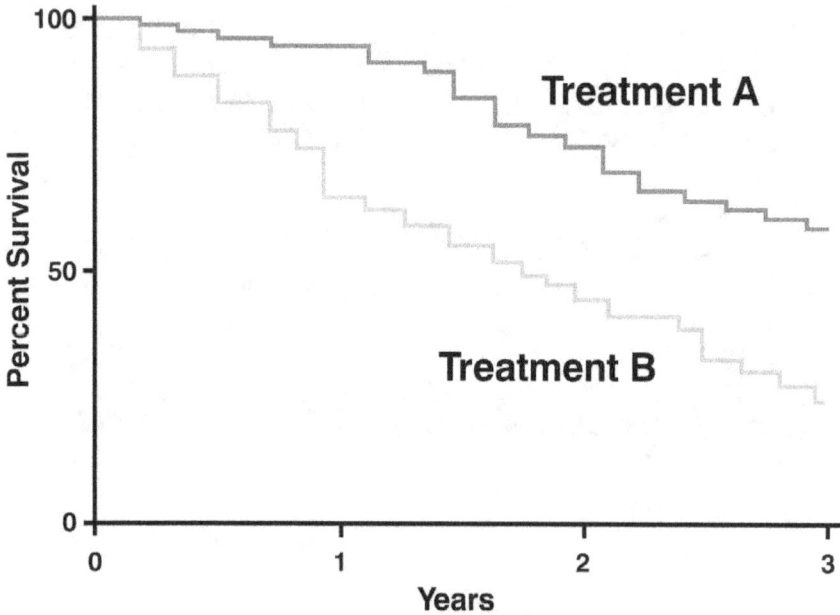

Fig 13. Kaplan-Meier plot

An important advantage of Kaplan–Meier plots is that they take into account censored data, which occurs if a patient withdraws from a study, is lost to follow-up, or is alive without event occurrence at last follow-up. On the plot, small vertical tick-marks indicate individual patients whose survival times have been censored. These patients contribute information until the point in time when they are censored (the tick), but are removed from the denominator thereafter.

PLOTS – QUIZ

QUESTIONS

Q1. Which type of statistical plot acts as a visual aid when communicating the risks and benefits of treatments to patients?

A. L'Abbe plots
B. Cates plot
C. Box and whiskers plot
D. Funnel plot
E. Forest plot

Q2. Which of the following statements regarding L'Abbe plots is FALSE?

A. They can be used to visually display data from meta-analysis
B. Treatment group results are plotted on the horizontal axis
C. They are a type of scatter-plot
D. Data on the upper left side of the plot indicates that experimental treatment is better than the control
E. The size of the trial is reflected by the size of the circle used

Q3. Which of the following statements regarding forest plots is true?

A. The area of the squares is inversely proportional to the number of events in each study
B. The length of the horizontal lines emerging from the squares represents the standard deviation
C. The meta-analysed measure of effect is plotted as a square
D. Larger studies are associated with smaller horizontal lines
E. Each study in the meta-analysis is represented by a diamond

Q4. Which of the following statements is true regarding box and whisker plots?

A. They are used to display qualitative variables
B. The box represents 25% of the data
C. Outliers cannot be plotted
D. The box is divided by the mode
E. 25% of the values lie below the lower quartile

ANSWERS

Q1. B. Cates plot

Q2. B. Treatment group results are plotted on the horizontal axis

Q3. D. Larger studies are associated with smaller horizontal lines

Q4. E. 25% of the data lie below the lower quartile

THE CONSORT GROUP

What is the CONSORT group?

CONSORT is an acronym for Consolidated Standards Of Reporting Trials. The CONSORT group is an international group of trialists, methodologists and medical journal editors. The main goal of the CONSORT group is to improve the reporting of randomized controlled trials by encouraging complete transparency from authors. Further information about the CONSORT group can be found at: www.consort-statement.org

The CONSORT statement

The CONSORT statement is an evidence-based, minimum set of recommendations for reporting randomized-controlled trials. It provides a standardized and reproducible means of reporting trial findings and enables readers to understand trail design, conduct, analysis and interpretation. It also assists with the assessment of the validity of the trials results.

The CONSORT statement consists of a 25-item checklist and the CONSORT flow diagram. The checklist does not need to be memorized but we have included it here as a point of reference. The consort checklist is actually an excellent way to help with the planning of a trial and writing a trial protocol. In any trial that is being conducted it is worthwhile to go through this list beforehand, rather than afterwards:

Title and Abstract:

1a. Identification as a randomized trial in the title.
1b. Structured summary of trial design, methods, results, and conclusions

Introduction:

2a. Scientific background and explanation of rationale
2b. Specific objectives or hypotheses

Methods:

3a. Description of trial design (such as parallel, factorial) including allocation ratio
3b. Important changes to methods after trial commencement (such as eligibility criteria), with reasons
4a. Eligibility criteria for participants
4b. Settings and locations where the data were collected
5. The interventions for each group with sufficient details to allow replication, including how and when they were actually administered
6a. Completely defined pre-specified primary and secondary outcome measures, including how and when they were assessed
6b. Any changes to trial outcomes after the trial commenced, with reasons
7a. How sample size was determined
7b. When applicable, explanation of any interim analyses and stopping guidelines
8a. Method used to generate the random allocation sequence
8b. Type of randomization; details of any restriction (such as blocking and block size)
9. Mechanism used to implement the random allocation sequence (such as sequentially numbered containers), describing any steps taken to conceal the sequence until interventions were assigned
10. Who generated the random allocation sequence, who enrolled participants, and who assigned participants to interventions
11a. If done, who was blinded after assignment to interventions (for example, participants, care providers, those assessing outcomes) and how
11b. If relevant, description of the similarity of interventions
12a. Statistical methods used to compare groups for primary and secondary outcomes
12b. Methods for additional analyses, such as subgroup analyses and adjusted analyses

Results:

13a. For each group, the numbers of participants who were randomly assigned, received intended treatment, and were analyzed for the primary outcome

13b. For each group, losses and exclusions after randomization, together with reasons

14a. Dates defining the periods of recruitment and follow-up

14b. Why the trial ended or was stopped

15. A table showing baseline demographic and clinical characteristics for each group

16. For each group, number of participants (denominator) included in each analysis and whether the analysis was by original assigned groups

17a. For each primary and secondary outcome, results for each group, and the estimated effect size and its precision (such as 95% confidence interval)

17b. For binary outcomes, presentation of both absolute and relative effect sizes is recommended

18. Results of any other analyses performed, including subgroup analyses and adjusted analyses, distinguishing pre-specified from exploratory

19. All important harms or unintended effects in each group

Discussion:

20. Trial limitations, addressing sources of potential bias, imprecision, and, if relevant, multiplicity of analyses

21. Generalizability (external validity, applicability) of the trial findings

22. Interpretation consistent with results, balancing benefits and harms, and considering other relevant evidence

Other information:

23. Registration number and name of trial registry

24. Where the full trial protocol can be accessed, if available

25. Sources of funding and other support (such as supply of drugs), role of funders

The CONSORT flow diagram

The CONSORT flow diagram is a flow diagram that depicts the passage of participants through a randomized controlled trial. The diagram explicitly shows the number of participants for each intervention group that was included in the primary data analysis. It is considered to improve the quality of randomized controlled trial reports and should show all exclusions and losses explicitly, with full explanation and reasoning for them.

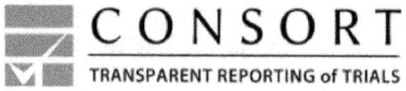

CONSORT 2010 Flow Diagram

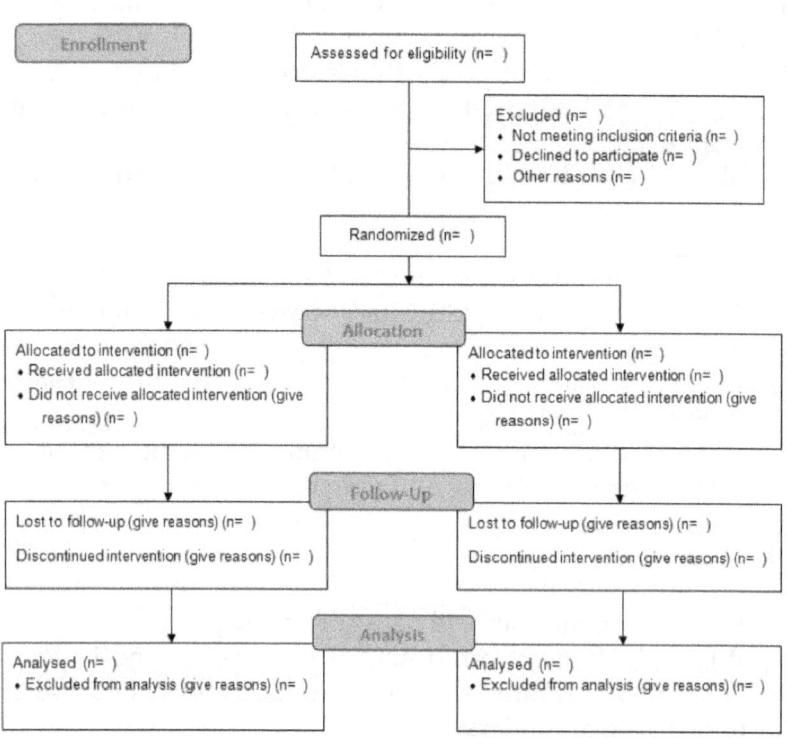

Fig 14. The CONSORT flow diagram template

THE CONSORT GROUP - QUIZ

QUESTIONS

Q1. How many items does the CONSORT statement checklist comprise?

A. 5
B. 10
C. 15
D. 20
E. 25

Q2. Which of the following statements regarding the CONSORT flow diagram is FALSE?

A. It should include a description of the trial methodology
B. It depicts the passage of participants through a randomized controlled trial
C. It explicitly shows the number of participants for each intervention group that was included in the primary data analysis
D. It is considered to improve the quality of randomized controlled trial reports
E. It should show all exclusions and losses explicitly

ANSWERS

Q1. E. 25

Q2. A. It should include a description of the trial methodology

LEVELS OF EVIDENCE & GRADING SYSTEMS

Levels of evidence

A hierarchical system of classifying evidence is an essential part of evidence-based medicine. This hierarchy is commonly referred to as the levels of evidence. When attempting to find the answer to a clinical conundrum a clinician should actively seek out papers with the highest level of evidence.

The term 'levels of evidence' was first used in a report by the Canadian Task Force on the Periodic Health Examination in 1979. The intention was to *grade the effectiveness of an intervention according to the quality of evidence obtained*. The Canadian Task Force originally described 4 levels of evidence:

LEVEL	TYPE OF EVIDENCE
I	At least 1 RCT with proper randomization
II.1	Well designed cohort or case-control study
II.2	Time series comparisons or dramatic results from uncontrolled studies
III	Expert opinions

Over the years many more grading systems have been described, some of the most commonly used being:

- Centre of Evidence-Based Medicine (CEBM), Oxford
- Strength-of-Recommendation Taxonomy (SORT)
- The Jadad scale
- Grading of Recommendations Assessment, Development and Evaluation (GRADE)

Centre of Evidence-Based Medicine

The Centre of Evidence-Based Medicine (CEBM) based at Oxford University is a not-for-profit organization that is dedicated to the practice, teaching and dissemination of high quality evidence-based medicine that was founded in 1995. The levels of evidence system developed by the CEBM has become one of the most widely used.

The CEBM levels of evidence are as follows:

LEVEL	TYPE OF EVIDENCE
1a	Systematic reviews (with homogeneity) of randomized controlled trials
1b	Individual randomized controlled trials (with narrow confidence intervals)
1c	All or none randomized controlled trials
2a	Systematic reviews (with homogeneity) of cohort studies
2b	Individual cohort studies or low quality randomized controlled trials (e.g. <80% follow-up)
2c	"Outcomes" research; ecological studies
3a	Systematic reviews (with homogeneity) of case-control studies
3b	Individual case-control study
4	Case series (and poor quality cohort and case-control studies)
5	Expert opinion, based on physiology, bench research or "first principles"

Strength-of-Recommendation Taxonomy

The Strength-of-Recommendation Taxonomy (SORT) is another popular system that was developed by the American Academy of Family Physicians. This system emphasizes the use of patient-orientated outcomes that measure changes in morbidity or mortality.

The SORT levels of evidence (codes) are as follows:

CODE	DEFINITION
A	Consistent, good-quality patient orientated evidence
B	Inconsistent or limited-quality patient orientated evidence
C	Consensus, disease-orientated evidence (often expert opinion or case series)

The Jadad scale

The Jadad scale, also known as the Oxford quality scoring system, is a means of assessing the quality of the methodology of a clinical trial. The scale is used for a variety of purposes including:

- To assist with critical appraisal of papers
- As a means of evaluating the quality of a paper
- As an inclusion criterion for including papers in a meta-analysis

The Jadad scale is widely accepted as being a simple and easy to use method for evaluating study methodology. It is considered to be reliable and an excellent means for identifying bias.

The Jadad scale consists of five questions, which are scored as follows:

1. Was the study described as randomized? (+1 Point)
2. Was the study described as double blind? (+1 Point)

3. Was there a description of withdrawals and dropouts? (+1 Point)
4. Was the method of randomization described and appropriate? (+1 Point)
5. Was the method of blinding described and appropriate? (+1 Point)

Points are deducted if:

1. The method used to generate the sequence of randomization was described and it was inappropriate. (-1 Point)
2. The study was described as double blind but the method of blinding was inappropriate. (-1 Point)

The Jadad scale has received criticism for being too simplistic and placing too much emphasis on blinding. It has also been shown to have a high degree of inconsistency between different raters. Another major criticism is that it does not take into account allocation concealment, which is considered to be of paramount importance by The Cochrane Collaboration.

Grading of Recommendations Assessment, Development and Evaluation (GRADE)

The Grading of Recommendations Assessment, Development and Evaluation (GRADE) working group was founded in 2000 as an informal collaboration of people with an interest in addressing the shortcomings of the present grading systems used in health care.

The GRADE approach is a method of assessing the certainty in evidence and the strength of recommendations in healthcare. It provides a structured and transparent evaluation of the importance of outcomes of alternative management strategies, acknowledgement of patients and the public values and preferences, and comprehensive criteria for downgrading and upgrading certainty in evidence.

The GRADE approach is summarized below:

LEVEL	QUALITY OF EVIDENCE	DEFINITION
A	High	Further research is very unlikely to change our confidence in the estimate of effect: • Several high-quality studies with consistent results • In special cases: one large, high-quality multi-centre trial
B	Moderate	Further research is likely to have an important impact on our confidence in the estimate of effect and may change the estimate: • One high-quality study • Several studies with some limitations
C	Low	Further research is very likely to have an important impact on our confidence in the estimate of effect and is likely to change the estimate: • One or more studies with severe limitations
D	Very Low	Any estimate of effect is very uncertain: • Expert opinion • No direct research evidence • One or more studies with very severe limitations

LEVELS OF EVIDENCE & GRADING SYSTEMS - QUIZ

QUESTIONS

Q1. Which of the following represents the highest level of evidence?

A. Systematic reviews of cohort studies
B. Systematic review of randomized controlled trials
C. Systematic reviews of case-control studies
D. Expert opinion
E. Bench research

Q2. Which of the following represents the highest level of evidence?

A. Systematic reviews of cohort studies
B. Ecological studies
C. Systematic reviews of case-control studies
D. Low quality randomized controlled trials (with < 80% follow-up)
E. Bench research

Q3. By which name is the Jadad scale also known?

A. Cardiff quality scoring system
B. Cambridge quality scoring system
C. Oxford quality scoring system
D. Edinburgh quality scoring system
E. London quality scoring system

Q4. Which of the following is NOT considered to be an advantage of the Jadad scale?

A. It provides an inclusion criterion for including papers in a meta-analysis
B. It can assist with critical appraisal of papers
C. It provides a simple and easy to use method for evaluating study methodology
D. It takes into account allocation concealment
E. It provides a reliable means for identifying bias

ANSWERS

Q1. B. Systematic review of randomized controlled trials

Q2. A. Systematic reviews of cohort studies

Q3. C. Oxford quality scoring system

Q4. D. It takes into account allocation concealment

SAMPLE DISTRIBUTION

Normal distribution

A normal distribution, also known as a Gaussian distribution, follows a classical bell shaped curve and is symmetrical around its mid-point. It is a continuous probability distribution.

The normal distribution is important because it is the distribution to which all possible distributions will converge if the sample size is large enough. If you take repeated samples to calculate, for example the average income in a population, each sample will by chance come up with a slightly different estimate of the mean income. If you then plotted the different means in a histogram you would notice that the distribution of these means will resemble a normal distribution, even if the original distribution of income in the population was not normal at all, e.g. highly skewed (e.g. most people having low income and some people having very high incomes). The larger the sample size of each of your samples, the more the distribution of the means will come resemble the normal distribution and will eventually completely converge to it.

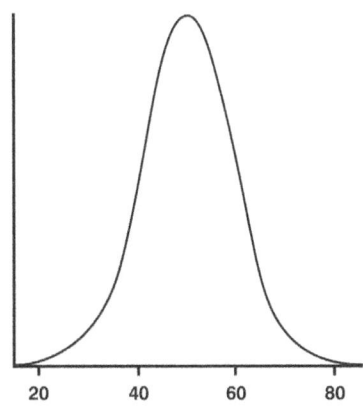

Fig 15. A normal, or Gaussian, distribution

In a normal distribution:

- The median is the middle point of the observations
- The mode is the most commonly observed measurement
- The mean is the arithmetic average

In a normal distribution the median = the mode = the mean.

Non-normal distributions do not have this symmetry property. They are generally skewed in one direction. The characteristics of a normal distribution do not apply if the distribution is skewed.

Positively skewed distribution

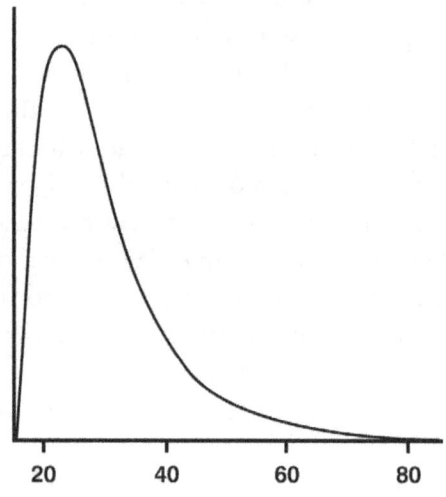

Fig 16. A positively skewed distribution

In a positively skewed distribution the tail of the graph lies in the positive direction (to the right).

In a positively skewed distribution the mean > the median > the mode.

In a positively skewed distribution the median is usually the preferred measurement.

Negatively skewed distribution

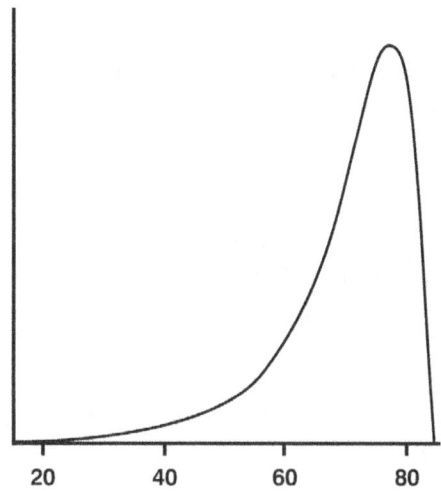

Fig 17. A negatively skewed distribution

In a negatively skewed distribution the tail of the graph lies in the negative direction (to the left).

In a negatively skewed distribution the mode > the median > the mean.

In a negatively skewed distribution the median is usually the preferred measurement.

SAMPLE DISTRIBUTION - QUIZ

QUESTIONS

Q1. Which of the following statements regarding Gaussian sample distribution is FALSE?

A. It can be skewed left or right
B. It is symmetrical around its mid-point
C. The mean is the arithmetic average
D. The median is the middle point of the observations
E. The mode is the most commonly observed measurement

Q2. Which of the following statements regarding sample distribution is true?

A. In a positively skewed distribution the mode is greater than the mean
B. The mode is the middle point of the observations
C. The median is the arithmetic average
D. In a skewed distribution the median is the preferred measurement
E. The mean is the most commonly observed measurement

Q3. Which of the following is true regarding positively skewed distributions?

A. The mean = median
B. The mode is the preferred measurement
C. The data is negatively skewed
D. The mode > mean
E. The mean > median

Q4. Which of the following is true regarding negatively skewed distributions?

A. The mean = median = mode
B. The median is the preferred measurement
C. The data is positively skewed
D. The mean > mode
E. The mean > median

ANSWERS

Q1. A. It can be skewed left or right

Q2. D. In a skewed distribution the median is the preferred measurement

Q3. E. The mean > median

Q4. B. The median is the preferred measurement

EPIDEMIOLOGICAL DATA

What is epidemiology?

Epidemiology is the study of the distribution and determinants of health-related states and events, including disease, and the application of this study to the control of disease. Epidemiology is a vitally important tool of evidence-based medicine as it helps to both identify risk factors for disease and to guide study design. Epidemiology itself uses statistics as a means to reach these two aims.

Prevalence

The prevalence is the proportion of individuals who have the disease at a given time point, usually the time of the interview. It does not include information on when the disease started or is likely to end. It is usually expressed as a percentage or fraction of the population. The main tool to measure prevalence is a cross sectional study. It should be noted that the time at which presence or absence of a condition is assessed usually varies among study participants, as it is usually impossible to assess all participants on a single day. A prevalence study may even intentionally span over a long time period with new participants being enrolled on a continuous basis, but each of them being assessed only once. This is often used in the case of seasonal conditions such as diarrhoea, resulting in an estimate of the average prevalence of the condition over that time period.

Prevalence is often used to describe conditions of long duration such as HIV infection, hypertension or diabetes. Conditions of short duration that are very common, such as diarrhoea or influenza-like illness may also be described by prevalence but diseases of short duration with a low probability of being present at a single point in time in an affected individual (e.g. meningitis or myocardial infarction) are difficult to describe as prevalence. Prevalence rates will be high in chronic conditions where recovery and death rates from that condition are low.

Prevalence can be expressed as:

- Point prevalence
- Period prevalence and;
- Lifetime prevalence

Point prevalence = <u>Number of people with a disease at a given time</u>
The size of the population at the same time

Period prevalence = Number of people with a disease at any
<u>time over a time period</u>
The size of the population over
that time period

Lifetime prevalence = The proportion of people that has
either had or has the disease within their lifetime

Incidence

There are two types of incidence: incidence risk (cumulative incidence) and incidence rate (sometimes called incidence density). Incidence can be assessed in cohort studies.

The incidence risk is the number of new cases of a disease occurring in a set time period (Usually annually). It is usually expressed as a fraction of the population at risk of developing the disease (e.g. per 1000 or per 100,000 of the population). Note that incidence risk and prevalence are both proportions, which means that similar statistical methods can be used to analyse them.

Incidence rate is the number of new cases over the total amount of person-time observed in a study. This measure accounts for the fact that in most studies the time an individual is observed varies among study participants. One participant may join the study initially and then drop out, while a second participant may join only later and remain in the study until the end. To calculate the total person time in a cohort study, one simply adds the time of observation of all individuals and uses this figure as the denominator.

Incidence risk = <u>Number of new cases over a defined time period</u>
Population size

Incidence rate = <u>Number of new cases over the study period</u>
Total person time observed in the study

Mortality rates

The mortality rate is a type of incidence that expresses the risk of death in a specified population over a set period of time:

Mortality rate = <u>Number of deaths over a defined time period</u>
Population size

When the mortality rate has been adjusted to take into account the presence of a confounding factor (for example age or gender) then it is referred to as the standardized mortality rate. Standardization is necessary to make two populations comparable. The classic example is the comparison of mortality in Alaska (which has relatively young population) with that of Florida (which has a lot of pensioners). Standardization is done by stratifying the population (e.g. that of Alaska) according to age groups and gender, calculating the mortality in each gender/age stratum and then allocating different weighting to each stratum according to the size of a standard population (e.g. the whole of the US), or a separate subpopulation (e.g. Florida). This then allows comparability of two populations.

The standardized mortality ratio is a ratio that quantifies an increase or decrease in the mortality of a cohort with respect to the general population.

EPIDEMIOLOGICAL DATA - QUIZ

QUESTIONS

Q1. A diabetic nurse screens 300 patients on a practice diabetic register as part of a health promotion exercise. She discovers that 75 of these patients have evidence of peripheral neuropathy. Based on this information which of the following statements is true?

A. The prevalence of peripheral neuropathy in the UK diabetic population is 25%
B. The prevalence of peripheral neuropathy in the practice diabetic population is 25%
C. The incidence of peripheral neuropathy in the UK diabetic population is 25%
D. The incidence of peripheral neuropathy in your the diabetic population is 25%
E. Further information is needed in order to calculate prevalence of peripheral neuropathy in this population

Q2. An audit looking at the incidence and prevalence of type 2 diabetes in a GP practice has been completed. In the year there have been 12 new cases diagnosed. There are currently 200 patients on the practice register with type 2 diabetes and your list size is 4000 patients. Based on this information which of the following statements is true?

A. The incidence and prevalence cannot be calculated from this audit
B. The incidence is 3%
C. The prevalence is 5%
D. The incidence is 5%
E. The prevalence is 0.3%

ANSWERS

Q1. B. The prevalence of peripheral neuropathy in the practice diabetic population is 25%

Q2. C. The prevalence is 5%

MEASURING DATA

What is data?

Data is any set of values that can be measured upon a scale. Data can be collected, measured, reported on and analyzed. It can also be visualized using a variety of different plots or graphs.

Data can be considered to be either:

- Categorical or;
- Quantitative

Categorical data

Categorical data is any statistical data type that consists of categorical variables. Their properties can be observed but cannot generally be measured easily in numerical terms.

Categorical data can be measured on either:

- A nominal scale or;
- An ordinal scale

The nominal scale is used to differentiate between items or characteristics in a descriptive manner. The assigned categories have no intrinsic order and bear no mathematical relationship with each other. Examples of data that is measured on a nominal scale are gender and hair color.

The ordinal scale is used to differentiate between items or characteristics that do not have a numerical value but do have an intrinsic order or ranking. Examples of data that is measured on an ordinal scale are social class and the position of an athlete in a race.

Nominal and ordinal data are analyzed using non-parametric statistics.

Quantitative data

Quantitative data is any statistical data type that can be measured on a numerical scale.

Quantitative data can be measured on either:

- An interval scale or;
- A ratio scale

Interval scales allow for the degree of difference between points on the scale but not the ratio between the points. Interval data has no true starting point and the value zero is set arbitrarily. Examples of data measured on an interval scale would be temperature on the Celsius scale and date when measured from a set era, e.g. AD.

Ratio scales are similar to interval scales but they have a true zero value. Examples of data type measured on a ratio scale are length, height and weight.

Interval and ratio data are usually analyzed using parametric statistics. However, sometimes non-parametric methods are used if the assumptions of a parametric test are not met.

MEASURING DATA - QUIZ

QUESTIONS

Q1. Which of the following types of data is measured on a nominal scale?

A. Position in a race
B. Social class
C. Gender
D. Height
E. Temperature in Celsius

Q2. Which of the following types of data is measured on an ordinal scale?

A. Date when measured from a set era, e.g. AD
B. Social class
C. Gender
D. Weight
E. Temperature in Fahrenheit

Q3. Which of the following types of data is measured on an interval scale?

A. Position in a race
B. Length
C. Gender
D. Social class
E. Temperature in Celsius

Q4. Which of the following types of data is measured on a ratio scale?

A. Position in a race
B. Gender
C. Weight
D. Date when measured from a set era, e.g. AD
E. Temperature in Celsius

Q5. Which of the following statements regarding scales of measurement is FALSE?

A. The nominal scale is for mutually exclusive data
B. The nominal scale collects quantitative data.
C. The ordinal scale involves ranking of the variable.
D. The Fahrenheit scale is an example of an interval scale.
E. The ratio scale has a definition of zero.

ANSWERS

Q1. C. Gender

Q2. B. Social class

Q3. E. Temperature in Celsius

Q4. C. Weight

Q5. B. The nominal scale collects quantitative data

DESCRIBING DATA

Variance

The variance is a measure of the spread of the observations around the mean value. It can be defined as the average of the squared differences from the mean.

The variance is equal to the square of the standard deviation (σ^2).

Standard deviation (σ)

The standard deviation is a measure of how spread out the data is. It is equal to the square root of the variance:

$$\text{Standard Deviation } (\sigma) = \sqrt{\text{variance}}$$

SD can be reasonably considered to be approximately the average difference each observation in a sample lies from the sample mean; the smaller the value of σ, the more tightly the data are grouped.

Standard error of the mean (SEM)

The standard error of the mean is the standard deviation of the sample distribution. It is a measure of how precisely the sample mean approximates the population mean. It is equal to the standard deviation divided by the square root of the sample size:

$$\text{Standard Error Mean} = \frac{\text{Standard deviation}}{\sqrt{\text{sample size}}}$$

The SEM is directly proportional to the standard deviation and inversely proportional to the sample size. It therefore decreases as the sample size increases and increases as the sample size decreases. A larger sample provides more information and therefore a more precise estimate with a smaller standard error.

In conclusion, the standard deviation is a property of the study population, reflecting how individuals in that population naturally differ from each other. It is for the most part fixed for a given population. If different random samples of the same population are taken and the SD taken, it will roughly be similar across the different samples, independent of the size of the sample. In contrast, the SEM is a property of the study, reflecting how precise the estimate is. It will always decrease as the sample size of the study becomes larger.

Confidence intervals

The SEM can be used to construct confidence intervals. A confidence interval shows the precision of a result with reference to the whole population.

A 95% confidence interval is the range of values that has a 95% probability of encompassing the 'true' value.

In a normal distribution:

- Approximately 68% of the observations lie within ± 1 SD of the mean
- Approximately 95% of the observations lie within ± 2 SD of the mean
- Approximately 99% of the observations lie within ± 3 SD of the mean
- **Exactly 95% of the observations lie within ± 1.96 SD of the mean**

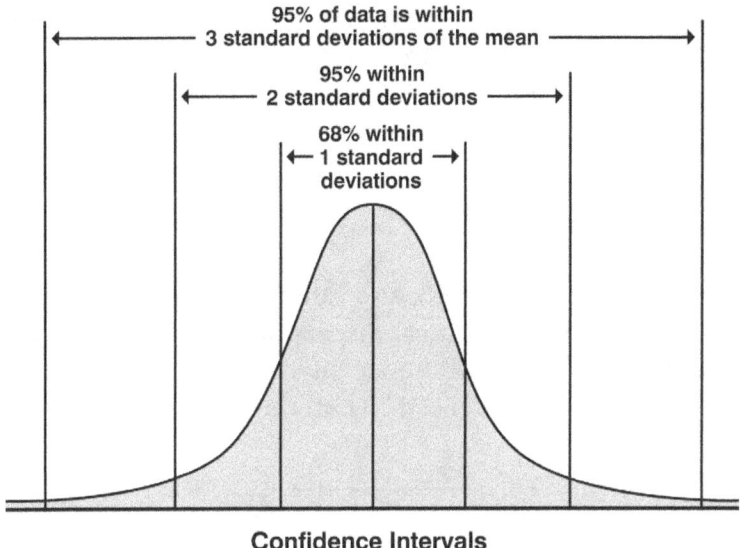

Confidence Intervals

Fig 18. Confidence intervals

The co-efficient of variation

The co-efficient of variation (CV) is the standard deviation of the data expressed as a percentage of the mean. It is useful when attempting to compare studies that have used different units to describe their data.

The co-efficient of variation is equal to the standard deviation divided by the mean multiplied by 100:

Co-efficient of variation = Standard deviation x 100
                                            Mean

Range

The range of a set of data is the difference between the highest and lowest values in the set. To find the range the data needs to be organized from smallest to the largest. Then subtract the smallest value from the largest value in the set.

Range is a simple and useful means for describing non-normally data but loses value if there are outlying values that fall far outside the rest of the data set.

Interquartile range

The interquartile range (IQR), also called the midspread or middle fifty, is a measure of statistical dispersion. It is the data that that lies between the lower and upper quartiles (25th and 75th centiles) and is therefore not influenced by outlying values:

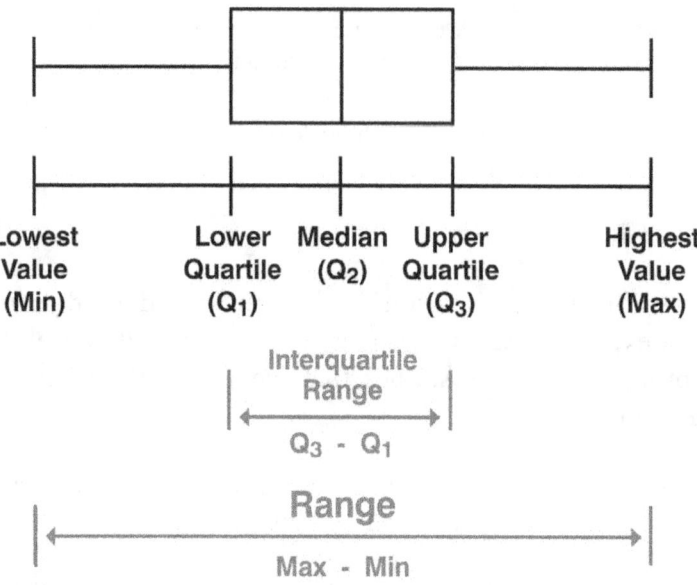

Fig 19. The interquartile range

Percentiles

A percentile, also known as a centile, is a measure used that indicates the value below which a given percentage of observations in a group of observations fall.

For example:

- The 20th percentile is the value below which 20% of the observations may be found
- The 50th percentile (which is equal to the median) is the value below which 50% of the observations may be found
- The 90th percentile is the value below which 90% of the observations may be found

DESCRIBING DATA - QUIZ

QUESTIONS

Q1. Which of the following statements regarding the standard error of the mean (SEM) is true? Select ONE answer only.

A. It increases as the sample size increases
B. It can be used to construct confidence intervals
C. A smaller sample provides a more precise estimate
D. It is inversely proportional to the standard deviation
E. It depends upon only the size of the sample

Q2. Which of the following statements regarding variance is true?

A. Variance can apply to skewed distributions
B. The standard deviation = 1 / variance
C. In a normal distribution 95% of the values lie within +/- 1.5 standard error of the mean
D. The standard error of the mean is a measure of how precisely the sample mean approximates the population mean
E. The larger the standard deviation the more tightly grouped the values

Q3. Which of the following statements regarding variance is FALSE?

A. The variance is a measure of the spread of the observations around the mean value.
B. Variance only applies to normally distributed data
C. The standard error increases with increasing sample size
D. The interquartile range lies between the 25th and the 75th centiles
E. In a normal distribution approximately 68% of the observation lie within +/- 1 standard deviation of the mean

Q4. Which of the following statements regarding standard deviation is true?

A. It is a measure of the spread of the sample distribution
B. It can be calculated from the square of the variance
C. It is a measure of how precisely the sample mean approximates the population mean
D. It is derived from the p value
E. It can be calculated by (variance / n^2), where n is the sample size

Q5. Which of the following statements is true regarding box and whisker plots?

A. They are used to display qualitative variables
B. The box represents 25% of the data
C. Outliers cannot be plotted
D. The box is divided by the mode
E. 25% of the values lie below the lower quartile

Q6. Which of the following statements is true regarding box and whisker plots?

A. They are used to display data that has a normal distribution
B. They are used to display qualitative variables
C. The box is divided by the mean
D. The box represents 50% of the data
E. 75% of the values lie above the upper quartile

ANSWERS

Q1. B. It can be used to construct confidence intervals

Q2. D. The standard error of the mean is a measure of how precisely the sample mean approximates the population mean

Q3. C. The standard error increases with increasing sample size

Q4. A. It is a measure of the spread of the sample distribution

Q5. E. 25% of the data lie below the lower quartile

Q6. D. The box represents 50% of the data

COMPARING DATA

Statistical tests

Data can be compared using a variety of different statistical tests. The choice of test depends upon the type of data being analyzed, the number of groups being compared and whether the data is paired or unpaired.

Nominal and ordinal data are analyzed using non-parametric statistical tests. Interval and ratio data are analyzed using parametric statistical tests.

When two groups of data are being compared the following statistical tests can be used:

	PARAMETRIC	NON-PARAMETRIC
PAIRED DATA	Paired students t-test	Wilcoxon signed-rank test
UNPAIRED DATA	Unpaired students t-test	Mann-Whitney U test

When three or more groups of data are being compared the following statistical tests can be used:

	PARAMETRIC	NON-PARAMETRIC
PAIRED DATA	Repeated measures ANOVA	Friedman test
UNPAIRED DATA	One-way ANOVA	Kruskall-Wallis test

When two proportions or percentages are being compared (for example in a 2 by 2 table) the following statistical tests can be used:

	SMALL SAMPLE	LARGE SAMPLE
PAIRED DATA	McNemar's test	McNemar's test
UNPAIRED DATA	Fisher's exact test	Chi-squared test

There are many other statistical tests in routine use. Simple survival curves such as those displayed by a Kaplan Meyer plot are compared using the log-rank test.

It should be noted that most of these tests do not give an effect estimate or confidence interval; instead all they usually do is provide a p-value.

The null hypothesis

The null hypothesis states that there is no significant difference between specified populations, any observed difference being due to sampling error.

The null hypothesis represents a theory that a new treatment would be no better, on average, than a current one. There is, in essence, no significant difference between the two treatments or groups. The aim of most studies is to disprove the null hypothesis.

The p-value

The p-value is the probability of rejecting the null hypothesis when the null hypothesis is true. The p-value depends on the sample size and the size of the difference between two groups. The larger the difference (effect size) and the larger the sample size, the smaller the p-value.

If the p-value is less than a pre-determined significance level (usually < 0.05) then the null hypothesis can be rejected and it can be assumed that the result is statistically significant.

Type I errors

A type I error is the incorrect rejection of the null hypothesis when it is true. For example, if a new drug is being tested, the null hypothesis would state that the new drug is no better, on average, than the current drug. A type I error occurs if it is concluded that the two drugs produce different effects, when in fact there was no difference between them.

The p-value is the estimated probability of rejecting the null hypothesis and therefore reflects type I error. The p-value is misleadingly low with a type I error.

Type II errors

A type II error is the acceptance of the null hypothesis when it is false. For example, if a new drug is being tested, the null hypothesis would state that the new drug is no better, on average, than the current drug. A type II error occurs if it is concluded that the two drugs have the same effect when in fact they produce different effects. It is most common for a type II error to occur in situations where the sample size is small.

When a type II error has occurred the p-value will be misleadingly high.

Alpha and beta

Alpha is the probability of making a type I error and beta is the probability of making a type II error.

Power

The power of a test measures the test's ability to make a correct decision, i.e. to reject the null hypothesis when it is incorrect. This equates to the probability of not committing a type II error. The maximum power a test can have is 1, and the minimum is 0.

The power of a study defines its ability to demonstrate an association between two variables if one actually exists. Power is equal to 1 – beta.

Z-scores

The z-score, also known as the standard score, indicates how many standard deviations a result is from the mean. If the z-score is 0 then the result is equal to the mean. If the z-score is greater than 2.2 (> 2.2 standard deviations greater than the mean) then the null hypothesis can be rejected.

COMPARING DATA - QUIZ

QUESTIONS

Q1. Which of the following is a non-parametric statistical test that can be used to compare two groups of paired data?

A. Paired students t-test
B. Wilcoxon signed-rank test
C. One-way ANOVA
D. Chi-squared test
E. Fisher's exact test

Q2. Which of the following is a non-parametric statistical test that can be used to compare five groups of unpaired data?

A. Unpaired students t-test
B. Friedman test
C. One-way ANOVA
D. Chi-squared test
E. Mann-Whitney U test

Q3. Which of the following statements regarding the null hypothesis is true?

A. The null hypothesis states that there is always a difference between the two groups
B. A type I error occurs when the null hypothesis has been accepted when it is actually false
C. The smaller the p value the less significant the result
D. The p value is misleadingly high with a type II error
E. If the Z-score is greater than 2.2 then the null hypothesis can be accepted

Q4. Which of the following statements regarding p-values is true?

A. The p value is considered statistically significant when it is less than 0.5
B. A p-value of 0.01 has a lower degree of statistical significance than a p-value of 0.05
C. The p-value is the probability of rejecting the null hypothesis when the null hypothesis is true
D. It reflects type II error
E. When a type I error has occurred the p-value will be misleadingly high

Q5. Which of the following statements regarding type I and type II errors is FALSE?

A. A type 1 error is the incorrect rejection of the null hypothesis when it is true
B. A type 2 error is the acceptance of the null hypothesis when it is false
C. When a type II error has occurred the p-value will be misleadingly high
D. A type 1 error occurs if it is concluded that the two drugs produce different effects, when in fact there was no difference between them
E. Alpha is the probability of making a type II error

ANSWERS

Q1. B. Wilcoxon signed-rank test

Q2. C. One-way ANOVA

Q3. D. The p value is misleadingly high with a type II error

Q4. C. The p-value is the probability of rejecting the null hypothesis when the null hypothesis is true

Q5. E. Alpha is the probability of making a type II error

CORRELATION & REGRESSION

Correlation

Correlation in statistics is used to examine the relationship between two quantitative variables. It is used in two main ways:

1. To examine the strength of the relationship
2. To examine whether the relationship is positive or negative

If the data is plotted on a scatterplot a correlation co-efficient can be used to quantify the relationship between the two variables.

In statistics three types of correlation co-efficient exist:

- Pearson's correlation co-efficient
- Kendall rank correlation
- Spearman correlation

Pearson's correlation co-efficient

Pearson's correlation co-efficient is used to measure the degree of relationship between linear related variables. It is a parametric measure and can only be used if a linear relationship exists and at least one of the variables is normally distributed.

Pearson's correlation coefficient is denoted by r and indicates how closely the plotted points lie to the line, r always takes a value between -1 and +1:

- When r is positive there is a positive correlation
- When r is negative there is a negative correlation
- When r is zero there is no correlation between the variables

The closer r is to zero the less the linear association between the variables. Values of -1 or +1 imply a perfect linear correlation between the variables. Correlation coefficients do not given information about the size of the increase or decrease and do not give a measure of agreement.

The degree of correlation is quantified as follows:

- High correlation = +0.5-1.0 or -0.5-1.0
- Medium correlation = +0.3-0.5 or -0.3-0.5
- Low correlation = +0.1-0.3 or -0.1-0.3

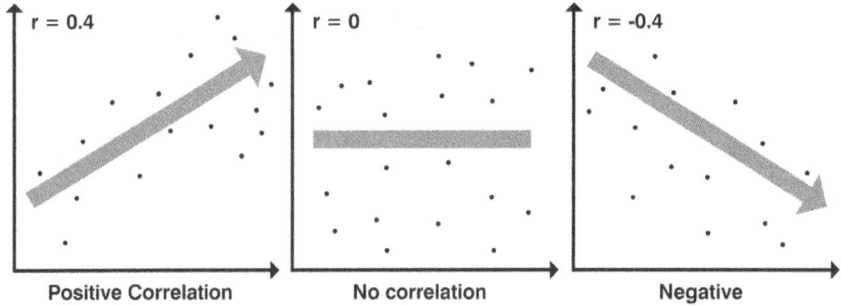

Fig 20. Scatterplots demonstrating positive and negative correlation

Kendall rank correlation

Kendall rank correlation, also known as the tau (τ) test, is a non-parametric test that measures the strength of dependence between the two variables. The calculations are based upon concordant and discordant pairs.

Spearman's rank correlation

Spearman's rank correlation, which is often denoted by rho (ρ), is a non-parametric test that measures the degree of association between the two variables.

Spearman's rank correlation test does not make any assumptions about the distribution of the data and is the appropriate correlation analysis when the variables are measured on a scale that is at least ordinal.

Regression analysis

Regression analysis can be used to estimate the relationship between variables. A linear regression line can be plotted using the regression equation. The slope and intercept of this line reflects the line that minimizes the summed-up differences from each data point to the line (more precisely, the squared differences).

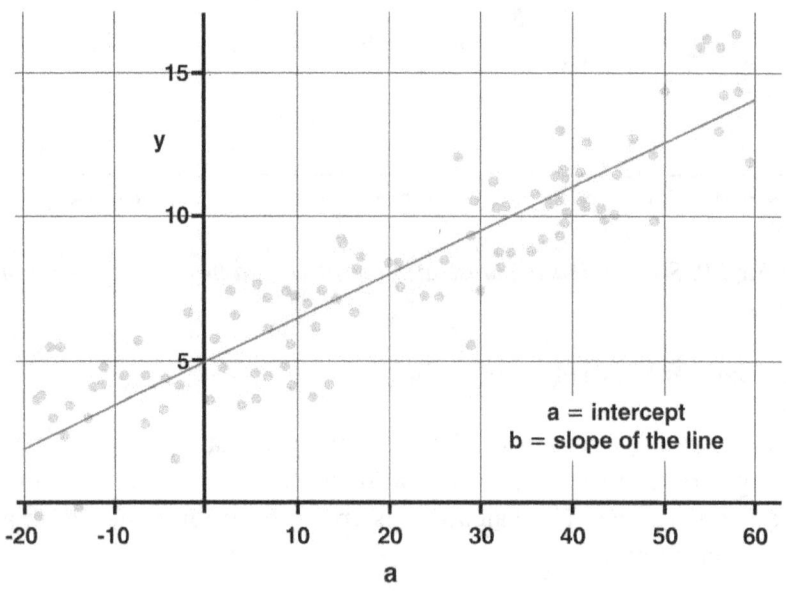

Fig 21. A linear regression line

When there is one independent variable the regression equation states that:

$$Y = a + bX$$

Where:

- a = the intercept (the value y takes when x is zero)
- b = the slope of the line (regression coefficient)
- Y = vertical axis
- X = horizontal axis

Therefore for any given value of X a corresponding value of Y can be predicted and vice versa. This process is called linear regression analysis.

In multivariable linear regression analysis, additional variables are added to the regression formula, and a separate slope can be calculated for each variable. The cloud of dots that can be seen in the scatterplot then becomes a multidimensional cloud, and again a line is fitted through this multidimensional cloud that minimizes the squared differences from each dot to the line.

Special statistical techniques have been developed to deal with outcomes (the Y in the equation) that are not quantitative but binary (e.g. dead or alive). In this situation Y can only assume 0 or 1 and all dots are distributed along two horizontal lines at Y= 0 and Y= 1. One commonly used statistical model for binary outcomes is called logistic regression.

For survival data, an advanced model called the Cox regression model is commonly used. The shared advantage of all these models is that they allow adjustment for several confounders at the same time, without the need for arduous stratification. Furthermore, in contrast to stratification regression analysis they allow accounting for confounders that are quantitative, such as blood pressure or age.

All regression models come with a set of different assumptions that need to be met so that the analysis produces a valid result. The most important assumption of most regression types is that the effect is following a linear trend as shown in Figure 21. Most regression models require a relatively large sample size. There are ways around most of these assumptions/conditions at the cost of ever increasingly complex models that become hard to interpret. The key to regression analysis is to keep it simple.

CORRELATION & REGRESSION - QUIZ

QUESTIONS

Q1. Which of the following statements regarding correlation coefficients is true?

A. When r is positive there is a negative correlation
B. The closer r is to zero the greater the linear association between the variables
C. A value of -1 implies a perfect linear correlation between the variables
D. They give a measure of agreement
E. Pearson's r is a non-parametric correlation coefficient.

Q2. Which of the following statements regarding correlation coefficients is FALSE?

A. The correlation coefficient is used to measure the strength of linear dependence between two variables
B. When r is negative there is a negative correlation
C. When r is zero there is no correlation between the variables
D. A significant correlation implies cause and effect.
E. Kendall's s is a non-parametric correlation coefficient

Q3. A scatter-plot of two variables is shown below. Which of the following statements regarding this scatter-plot is true?

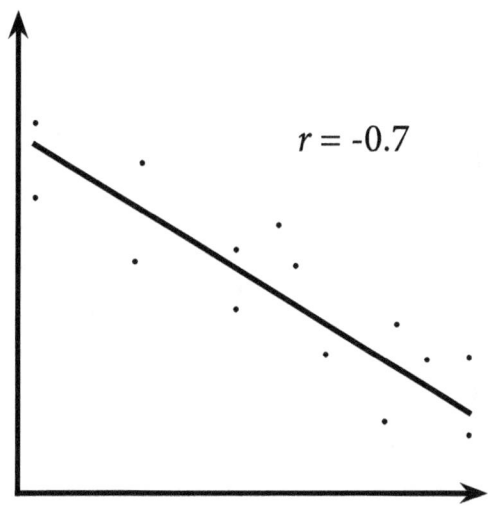

$r = -0.7$

A. There is no correlation between the two variables
B. There is a high positive correlation
C. There is a low negative correlation
D. The correlation implies cause and effect
E. There is a high negative correlation

Q4. A scatter-plot of two variables is shown below. Which of the following statements regarding this scatter-plot is most true?

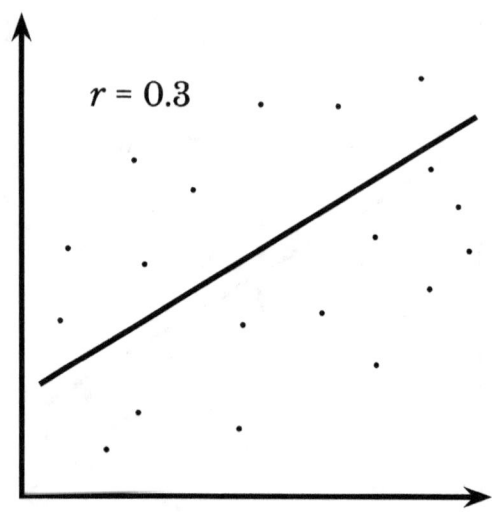

A. There is no correlation between the two variables
B. There is a low positive correlation
C. There is a high positive correlation
D. There is a low negative correlation
E. There is a high negative correlation

ANSWERS

Q1. C. A value of -1 implies a perfect linear correlation between the variables

Q2. D. A significant correlation implies cause and effect.

Q3. E. There is a high negative correlation

Q4. B. There is a low positive correlation

RISK & ODDS

Risk vs. odds

The terms 'risk' and 'odds' are often used interchangeably but they actually have quite different implications and are calculated in different ways.

Odds is a concept that is very familiar to gamblers. It is a ratio of probability that a particular event will occur and can be any number between zero and infinity. It is usually expressed as a ratio of two integers. For example an odds of 0.1 is written as 1:10 and an odds of 5 is written as 5:1.

Risk and risk ratios are more commonly used than odds and odds ratios in medicine as these are much more intuitive. Risk describes the probability of an event occurring. In medicine this is often an undesirable health outcome or adverse event. Risk is usually expressed as a number between zero and 1, although it can also be converted into a percentage. For example if there is 0.1 risk of developing a disease that means 1 in 10 people will develop the disease.

Odds and odds ratios rather than risk ratios are used in case-control studies because risks cannot be calculated. However, odds and odds ratios can also used to display the results of cross sectional studies, cohort studies and randomized controlled trials. The reason for this is that a commonly used regression model for binary (dichotomous) outcomes called logistic regression only allows the calculation of the odds ratio and not the risk ratio. Logistic regression models are fairly easy to do, and historically required little computing power. However, nowadays any smart phone has enough computing power to enable the use of regression models for binary data that can calculate the risk ratio (e.g. the log-binomial regression model).

Contingency tables

Contingency tables are a useful tool when attempting to calculate risk and make risk comparisons between different treatments being compared in a study.

Study results can be tabulated into a simple 2 x 2 contingency table as follows:

	DISEASE POSITIVE	DISEASE NEGATIVE
EXPERIMENTAL GROUP	A	B
CONTROL GROUP	C	D

This contingency table can then be used to calculate the control event rate (CER) and the experimental event rate (EER)

The EER is the event rate in the group given treatment with the experimental drug being investigated. This is also sometimes referred to as the absolute risk in the treatment group (ART).

The EER can be calculated from the above contingency table as follows:

$$EER = A \, / \, A + B$$

The CER is the event rate in the group given the control drug, which is sometimes a placebo. This is also sometimes referred to as the absolute risk in the control group (ARC).

The CER can be calculated from the above contingency table as follows:

$$CER = C \, / \, C + D$$

Relative risk

Relative risk (RR), which is also referred to as the risk ratio, is a ratio of the risk in each group. The relative risk is therefore a ratio of the EER and the CER:

$$RR = EER / CER$$

Absolute risk reduction

The absolute risk reduction (ARR) is the difference between the CER and the EER. The ARR can also be used to calculate the number needed to treat.

$$ARR = CER - EER$$

Relative risk reduction

The relative risk reduction (RRR) is the proportional reduction in the outcome rates between the experimental and control groups. It is calculated by dividing the ARR by the CER:

$$RRR = ARR / CER$$

The number needed to treat

The number needed to treat (NNT) is the average number of patients who need to be treated to prevent one additional adverse outcome. If a particular drug has a NNT of 5, it means that 5 people will have to be treated with this drug to prevent one additional adverse outcome. The ideal NNT is 1, where everyone that receives the treatment improves and no one improves with the control. The higher that the NNT is the less effective that the treatment is.

It is equal to the inverse of the ARR:

$$NNT = 1 / ARR$$

The number needed to harm

The number needed to harm (NNH) is calculated in the same way as the NNT but is used to describe adverse events. For NNH large values are considered favorable as this means that adverse events occur rarely. Conversely small values are considered to be unfavorable as this means that adverse events occur commonly.

Worked example

The best way to solidify an understanding of these concepts is to work through an example. Consider a study that has been performed to investigate a new treatment for preventing acute kidney injury in patients with diabetes mellitus.

A table showing the results of the study is shown below:

	Outcome: Developed acute kidney injury	Outcome: Normal renal function	Total patients
Drug X	100	900	1000
Placebo	200	800	1000
Total patients	300	1700	2000

In this study the CER can be calculated as follows:

$$CER = 200 / 1000$$
$$CER = 0.2$$

The EER can be calculated as follows:

$$EER = 100 / 1000$$
$$EER = 0.1$$

The RR can be calculated as follows:

$$RR = EER / CER$$
$$RR = 0.1 / 0.2$$
$$RR = 0.5$$

The ARR can be calculated as follows:

$$ARR = CER - EER$$
$$ARR = 0.2 - 0.1$$
$$ARR = 0.1$$

The RRR can be calculated as follows:

$$RRR = ARR / CER$$
$$RRR = 0.1 / 0.2$$
$$RRR = 0.5$$

The NNT can be calculated as follows:

$$NNT = 1 / ARR$$
$$NNT = 1 / 0.1$$
$$NNT = 10$$

RISK & ODDS - QUIZ

QUESTIONS

Q1. A study is carried out evaluating the relationship between omega 3 supplementation and myocardial infarction (MI) in men over the age of 65. The study examined the MI rate in 100 men taking omega 3 over a 2-year period and 100 men taking placebo over a 2-year period. Over the 2-year period 5 men in the omega 3 group suffered an MI, whereas 15 men in the placebo group suffered an MI. What is the relative risk of suffering a myocardial infarction?

A. 0.15
B. 0.03
C. 3.0
D. 0.33
E. 0.66

Q2. A cohort study is conducted to evaluate the relationship between dietary calcium supplementation and the occurrence of hip fractures in post-menopausal women. The study examines the hip fracture rate in 500 women taking calcium supplements and 500 women taking placebo over five years. Over the five-year period, 10 women have hip fractures in the calcium group and 25 women have hip fractures in the placebo group. What is the absolute risk reduction of a hip fracture?

A. 0.03
B. 0.3
C. 0.4
D. 15
E. None of the above

Q3. A study has been performed looking at a new treatment for preventing myocardial infarction in patients with diabetes mellitus. 1000 patients were treated with the new medication and 100 patients in this group went on to suffer a stroke. 1000 received no treatment and 200 patients in this group went on to suffer a stroke. Which of the following is the number needed to treat (NNT)?

A. 5
B. 10
C. 20
D. 50
E. 100

ANSWERS

Q1. D. 0.33

Q2. A. 0.03

Q3. B. 10

DIAGNOSTIC TESTS & SCREENING PROGRAMS

Diagnostic tests

A diagnostic test can be defined as '*any kind of medical test performed to aid in the diagnosis or detection of disease, injury or any other medical condition*'. Typically with any diagnostic test some of those at risk will be missed (false negatives) and some people not at risk will screen positive (false positives).

Diagnostic tests can be compared against a gold standard test to evaluate their usefulness. The gold standard test refers to a diagnostic test that is the most accurate and best available under reasonable conditions. An example of a gold standard test is a CT pulmonary angiogram for the diagnosis of a pulmonary embolus. Gold standard tests tend to change over time as medical science advances.

If the results of the diagnostic test are compared with the gold-standard test in a simple 2 x 2 table various useful statistical measures can be determined that assist in the evaluation of the diagnostic test:

	Disease positive with gold-standard test	Disease negative with gold standard test
Positive diagnostic test	A	B
Negative diagnostic test	C	D

Sensitivity

Sensitivity is the proportion of true positives correctly identified by the test. It can be calculated from the 2 x 2 table by the following formula:

$$\text{Sensitivity} = A / A + C$$

SeNsitivity is used to rule **OUT** a disease, and this can be remembered using the mnemonic **SNOUT**. It is a good indicator of the ability of a diagnostic test to detect a disease when it is present.

A value approaching 1 is desirable for ruling out a disease and indicates a low false-negative rate. Sensitivity is best used when screening for diseases with a low prevalence.

Specificity

The specificity is the proportion of true negatives correctly identified by the test. It can be calculated from the 2 x 2 table by the following formula:

$$\text{Specificity} = D / B + D$$

SPecificity is used to rule a disease **IN**, and this can be remembered using the mnemonic **SPIN**. It is a good indicator of the ability of a diagnostic test to confirm the absence of a disease when it is not present

A value approaching 1 is desirable for ruling a disease in and indicates a low false-positive rate.

Positive predictive value

The positive predictive value (PPV) is the proportion of those who test positive who actually have the disease. It can be calculated from the 2 x 2 table by the following formula:

$$\text{PPV} = A / A + B$$

It is the proportion of positive test results that are true positives and it represents the probability that a person that tests positive actually has the disease. It is affected by the prevalence of a disease and tests that have high sensitivity and specificity will have a low positive predictive value if the prevalence of the disease is low.

Negative predictive value

The negative predictive value (NPV) is the proportion of those who test negative who do not have the disease. It can be calculated from the 2 x 2 table by the following formula:

$$NPV = D / C + D$$

It is the proportion of negative test results that are true negatives and it represents the probability that a person that tests negative is actually disease free.

Like the positive predictive value, the negative predictive value is also dependant upon the prevalence of the disease, and will vary between populations.

Likelihood ratios

Likelihood ratios are another means of assessing the value of performing a diagnostic test. They are considered to be more useful than predictive values when determining whether a test result usefully changes the probability that a disease state is present. Because they are calculated from the sensitivity and specificity of the test they are independent of prevalence.

The likelihood ratio (LR+) for a positive test result can be calculated using the following formula:

$$LR + = \frac{sensitivity}{1 - specificity}$$

The likelihood ratio (LR-) for a negative test result can be calculated using the following formula:

$$LR- = \frac{1 - \text{sensitivity}}{\text{specificity}}$$

In summary, a likelihood ratio:

- Applies to a piece of diagnostic information
- Tells you how useful that information is when making a diagnosis
- Is a number between zero and infinity
- If greater than one, indicates that the information increases the likelihood of the suspected diagnosis
- If less than one, indicates that the information decreases the likelihood of the suspected diagnosis

Pre- and post-test probabilities

The pre-test probability is the proportion of people in the population who have the disease at a specific time or time interval. This is essentially the point prevalence or the period prevalence of the disease. Pre-test probabilities in medicine can be estimated using a clinician's judgment.

Post-test probability is the proportion of patients testing positive who truly have the disease. It is similar to the positive predictive value and represents the probability of the patient having a disease taking into account the results of the test.

The Fagan nomogram, also referred to as the likelihood ratio nomogram, can be used to determine the post-test probability by using the pre-test probability and the likelihood ratio.

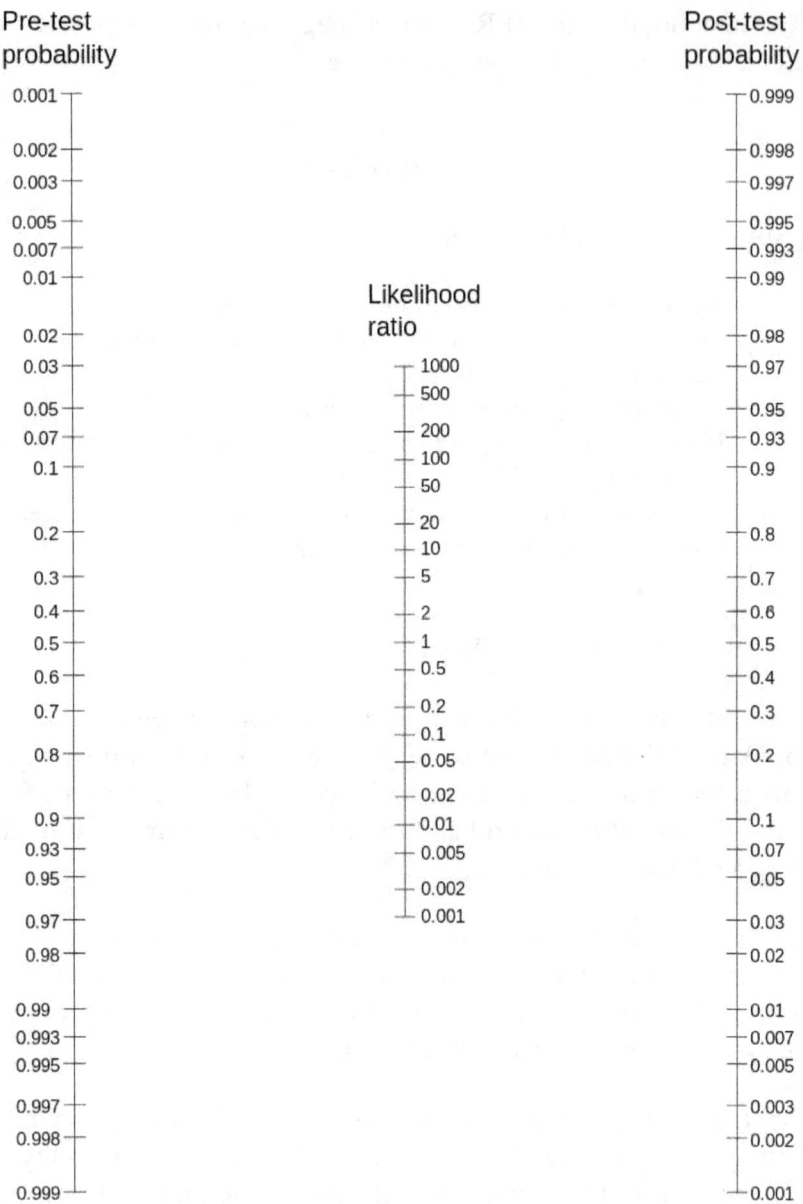

Fig 22. The Fagan nomogram

If a line is plotted connecting the pre-test probability and the calculated likelihood ratio it will intersect at the post-test probability on the right hand side of the Fagan nomogram.

Receiver operating characteristic curve

A receiver operating characteristic (ROC) curve is a graph used to assess diagnostic tests. The cut off point for a positive and negative test is varied and then the sensitivity and specificity for each of these cut off is calculated. A perfect test has a ROC curve that passes through the upper left corner (100% sensitivity, 100% specificity). Therefore the closer the ROC curve is to the upper left corner, the higher the overall accuracy of the test.

The area under the curve is a measure of how good the test is:

- 1 = perfect test
- 0.5 = test no better than chance

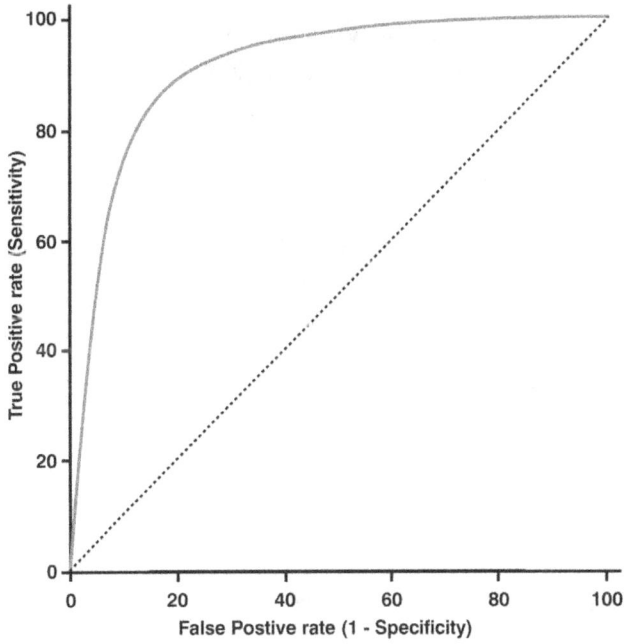

Fig 23. ROC curve

Worked example

Once again the best way to solidify an understanding of these concepts is to work through an example. Consider a new troponin assay that is being assessed on its ability to detect non-ST elevation myocardial infarction (NSTEMI). It was used in 1820 patients at 6 hours after the onset of chest pain. In patients with a positive troponin assay the presence of an NSTEMI was confirmed or refuted using angiography as the gold standard test.

The 2 by 2 table below displays the results:

	Positive angiogram	Negative angiogram
Positive troponin test	260	32
Negative troponin test	45	1483

The sensitivity can be calculated by:

$$\text{Sensitivity} = A / A + C$$
$$\text{Sensitivity} = 260 / (260 + 45)$$
$$\text{Sensitivity} = 0.85$$

The specificity can be calculated by:

$$\text{Specificity} = D / B + D$$
$$\text{Specificity} = 1483 / (1483 + 32)$$
$$\text{Specificity} = 0.98$$

The positive predictive value can be calculated by:

$$\text{PPV} = A / A + B$$
$$\text{PPV} = 260 / (260 + 32)$$
$$\text{PPV} = 0.89$$

The negative predictive can be calculated by:

$$\text{NPV} = D / C + D$$
$$\text{NPV} = 1483 / (45 + 1483)$$
$$\text{NPV} = 0.97$$

The likelihood ratio (LR+) for a positive test result can be calculated by:

$$LR+ = sensitivity / 1 - specificity$$
$$LR+ = 0.85 / (1 - 0.98)$$
$$LR+ = 42.5$$

The likelihood ratio (LR-) for a negative test result can be calculated by:

$$LR- = 1 - sensitivity / specificity$$
$$LR+ = (1 - 0.85) / 0.98$$
$$LR+ = 0.153$$

Screening tests

Screening tests are diagnostic tests used to identify individuals that have a disease of which they are unaware, before it develops or causes significant problems. They are therefore generally performed in apparently healthy individuals. This process can be more difficult and dangerous to the patient and to the healthcare systems sparse resources than one might think.

Screening programs

Screening programs are used as a means of identifying an unrecognized disease in individuals that are not yet exhibiting the clinical features of that disease. There are therefore generally performed in healthy individuals.

The aim of any screening program is the early identification of disease so that early treatment can be implemented. This may have the effect of reducing the morbidity and mortality of the disease whilst also reducing the financial burden of the disease upon the organization or institution responsible for its management. This is not, however, always the case.

Screening programs also have several associated problems including over-diagnosis, missed diagnosis and creation of adverse events associated with further investigation following a positive screening test.

The Wilson-Jungner criteria

The Wilson-Jungner criteria are one commonly quoted means of appraising the validity of a screening program.

The Wilson-Jungner criteria are as follows:

- The condition being screened for should be an important health problem
- The natural history of the condition should be well understood
- There should be a detectable early stage
- Treatment at an early stage should be of more benefit than at a later stage
- A suitable test should be devised for the early stage
- The test should be acceptable
- Intervals for repeating the test should be determined
- Adequate health service provision should be made for the extra clinical workload resulting from screening
- The risks, both physical and psychological, should be less than the benefits
- The costs should be balanced against the benefits

The ideal disease to be screened for is homocysteinuria. It is relatively common, well understood, and easy to diagnose by screening tests with high sensitivity and specificity. Confirmatory tests are also harmless to the patient. Early treatment before symptoms develop is crucial to prevent serious disease. Treatment is harmless as it simply entails adhering to a specific diet. In the highly unlikely event that a child is erroneously diagnosed with the condition, adverse effects of treatment would be minimal as the diet is not known to be harmful to those not afflicted by homocystinurea.

Contrast this with screening for breast cancer. The natural history of the disease is not well understood as it remains unclear what proportion of detected malignancy will eventually become invasive (perhaps only 10%). The diagnostic test used (mammography) may itself cause cancer. The sensitivity and specificity of mammography to detect breast cancer is relatively poor. Confirmatory tests (e.g. biopsy) are rather invasive. There is some benefit in early treatment, but this does not apply to all age groups (younger women appear to benefit less from early treatment than older women). Treatment is invasive (surgery) and toxic (radiotherapy and chemotherapy). Erroneously diagnosing a woman with a cancer that would never have killed her may have catastrophic consequences. For these reasons breast cancer screening remains a controversial screening program.

DIAGNOSTIC TESTS & SCREENING PROGRAMS - QUIZ

QUESTIONS

Q1. A study was performed on a group of 100 patients attending an Emergency Department review clinic with a possible scaphoid fracture. The aim was to evaluate the utility of ultrasound scanning in the diagnosis of scaphoid fracture. MRI was used to as the gold standard to confirm the diagnosis. Of the patients with a positive ultrasound scan 24 had a scaphoid fracture whilst 7 did not. Of the patients with a negative ultrasound scan 5 had a scaphoid fracture whilst 64 did not. Which of the following statements is true?

A. The sensitivity of ultrasound scanning for the diagnosis of a scaphoid fracture is 24/29
B. The specificity of a positive ultrasound scan for the diagnosis of a scaphoid fracture is: 64/69
C. The negative predictive value of ultrasound scanning in patients with possible scaphoid fracture is: 24/31
D. The positive predictive value of ultrasound scanning in patients with a possible scaphoid fracture is: 64/71
E. The specificity of ultrasound scanning is dependant upon the prevalence of scaphoid fracture in the test population.

Q2. A new D-dimer assay was used in 1430 patients to detect deep vein thrombosis (DVT) in patients with calf pain and/or swelling. In patients with a positive D-dimer the presence of a DVT was confirmed or refuted using doppler ultrasound scanning. The table below displays the results:

	DVT present	DVT not present
Positive d-dimer	436	32
Negative d-dimer	168	794

Which of the following statements is true?

A. The sensitivity of the D-dimer assay is 72%
B. The specificity of the D-dimer assay is 93%
C. The positive predictive value of the D-dimer assay is 82%
D. The negative predictive value of the D-dimer assay is 96%
E. The negative predictive value of the D-dimer assay is 72%

Q3. Which of the following statements regarding likelihood ratios (LRs) is FALSE?

A. The likelihood ratio for a positive test = sensitivity / (1-specificity)
B. The likelihood ratio for a negative test = (1-sensitivity) / specificity
C. They are a number between zero and infinity
D. If less than one, indicates that the information increases the likelihood of the suspected diagnosis
E. They apply to a piece of diagnostic information

Q4. Which of the following statements regarding the Wilson-Jungner criteria for appraising the validity of a screening programme is true?

A. The test can be used to understand the natural history of the condition
B. Treatment should be effective regardless of the disease stage
C. Intervals for repeating the test should be determined
D. There should be no extra clinical workload created as a consequence of the screening
E. Psychological risks need not be factored

ANSWERS

Q1. A. The sensitivity of ultrasound scanning for the diagnosis of a scaphoid fracture is 24/29

Q2. A. The sensitivity of the D-dimer assay is 72%

Q3. D. If less than one, indicates that the information increases the likelihood of the suspected diagnosis

Q4. C. Intervals for repeating the test should be determined

GLOSSARY OF TERMS

Absolute risk reduction:
The absolute risk reduction is the difference between the control event rate and the experimental event rate.

Allocation concealment:
Allocation concealment ensures that both clinicians and participants unaware of the treatment being allocated prior to enrollment in the study.

Alpha:
Alpha is the probability of making a type I error

Beta:
Beta is the probability of making a type II error.

Bias:
Bias is a systematic error in the way a trial is designed or run resulting in an inaccuracy in the result. There are numerous types of bias that can occur.

Case-control study:
A case-control study is a type of observational study in which two groups of patients, one with the disease and one without, are compared on the basis of a proposed causative factor that occurred in the past.

Clinical audit:
'A quality improvement process that seeks to improve patient care and outcomes through systematic review of care against explicit criteria and the implementation of change.'

Clinical drug trial:
A clinical drug trial is a study that is carefully designed to assess the benefits and risks of a specific investigational drug.

Clinical end-point:
A clinical end-point is a measurement of a direct clinical outcome. Examples of this would include mortality, morbidity, survival, improvements in quality of life or relief of symptoms.

Clinical governance:
'A system through which NHS organizations are accountable for continuously improving the quality of their services and safeguarding high standards of care by creating an environment in which excellence in clinical care will flourish.'

Cochrane Collaboration:
The Cochrane Collaboration is an independent organization that was formed to organize medical research information in a systematic way.

Co-efficient of variation:
The co-efficient of variation is the standard deviation of the data expressed as a percentage of the mean.

Cohort study:
A cohort study is a form of longitudinal, observational study that follows a group of patients (the cohort) forward in time to monitor the effects of a proposed etiological factor upon them.

Composite end-point:
Composite end-points combine a number of different measurements into a single composite end-point. These sorts of end-point are useful when any single event occurs too infrequently to be used as an end-point on its own.

Confidence interval:
A confidence interval shows the precision of a result with reference to the whole population.

Confounding factors:
Confounding factors are variables that have not been controlled or eliminated by the researcher. These variables differ between the two groups being studied and affect the outcome of interest.

Crossover study:
The crossover study is a modification of the randomized controlled trial, in which each patient receives both treatment and placebo in a random order.

Cross-sectional study:
A cross-sectional study is a type of observational study that involves collecting data at a set, defined time point.

Diagnostic test:
A diagnostic test is any kind of medical test performed to aid in the diagnosis or detection of disease, injury or any other medical condition.

End-point:
An end-point is an outcome or event that can be measured objectively to determine whether the intervention being studied is beneficial or not.

Epidemiology:
Epidemiology is the study of the distribution and determinants of health-related states and events, including disease, and the application of this study to the control of disease.

Evidence-based medicine:
Evidence-based medicine is the conscientious, explicit and judicious use of current best evidence in making decisions about the care of the individual patient. It means integrating individual clinical expertise with the best available external clinical evidence from systematic research.'

Experimental study:
Experimental studies are characterized by the fact that the study subjects are allocated by the investigator to the different study groups through the use of randomization.

External validity:
The external validity is the extent to which the results of a study can be extrapolated to other situations and to other people. Its is a measure of how the study findings apply to the wider population

Incidence:
The incidence is the rate of new cases of a disease occurring in a set time period.

Internal validity:
The internal validity of a study is the extent to which the methodology permits a conclusion about causal relationships to be made. It looks at whether the study methodology and design was of a suitable quality to avoid confounding.

Interquartile range:
The interquartile range (IQR) is the data that that lies between the lower and upper quartiles.

Meta-analysis:
Meta-analysis is a statistical procedure that integrates the results of multiple independent studies with common features with the goal of identifying patterns and variability amongst the study results.

Mortality rate:
The mortality rate is a type of incidence that expresses the risk of death in a specified population over a set period of time.

Negative predictive value:
The negative predictive value is the proportion of those who test negative who do not have the disease.

Normal distribution:
A normal distribution, also known as a Gaussian distribution, follows a classical bell shaped curve and is symmetrical around its mid-point. It is a continuous probability distribution.

Null hypothesis:
The null hypothesis is that there is no significant difference between specified populations, any observed difference being due to sampling or experimental error.

Number needed to treat:
The number needed to treat is the average number of patients who need to be treated to prevent one additional adverse outcome.

P-value:
The p-value is the probability of rejecting the null hypothesis when the null hypothesis is true.

Percentile:
A percentile is a measure used that indicates the value below which a given percentage of observations in a group of observations fall.

Positive predictive value:
The positive predictive value is the proportion of those who test positive who actually have the disease.

Post marketing surveillance:
Post-marketing surveillance (PMS) is the practice of monitoring the safety of a drug within the patient population after it has been released.

Power:
The power of a test measures the test's ability to make a correct decision, i.e. to reject the null hypothesis when it is incorrect. This equates to the probability of not committing a type II error.

Prevalence:
The prevalence is the actual number of cases of a disease at a set point in time.

Qualitative data:
Qualitative data is any statistical data type that consists of categorical variables. Their properties can be observed but cannot generally be measured easily in numerical terms.

Quantitative data:
Quantitative data is any statistical data type that can be measured on a numerical scale.

Randomization:
Randomization is the process by which an individual has an equal chance of entering any group within a study. It serves to reduce bias by distributing characteristics of patients that may influence outcomes randomly between the groups.

Relative risk:
Relative risk is a ratio of the risk in the experimental and control groups.

Relative risk reduction:
The relative risk reduction is the proportional reduction in the outcome rates between the experimental and control groups.

Screening test:
A screening test is a diagnostic test used to identify individuals that have a disease of which they are unaware, before it develops or causes significant problems.

Sensitivity:
Sensitivity is the proportion of true positives correctly identified by the test.

Specificity:
The specificity is the proportion of true negatives correctly identified by the test.

Standard deviation:
The standard deviation is a measure of how spread out the data is. It is equal to the square root of the variance:

Standard error of the mean:
The standard error of the mean is the standard deviation of the sample distribution. It is a measure of how precisely the sample mean approximates the population mean.

Surrogate end-point:
A surrogate end point is a measurement that may correlate with a clinical end-point but is not guaranteed to do so. An example of a surrogate end-point would be the measuring of gastric pH instead of the actual clinical end-point, which would be upper gastrointestinal bleeding.

Systematic review:
A systematic review looks at a particular research question and attempts to review systematically all of the pertinent articles relating to that question.

Type I error:
A type 1 error is the incorrect rejection of the null hypothesis when it is true.

Type II error:
A type 2 error is the acceptance of the null hypothesis when it is false.

Validity:
Validity is a means of measuring the end-points chosen by a study. It is the extent to which a conclusion, or measurement, is well founded and corresponds accurately to the real world.

Variance:
The variance is a measure of the spread of the observations around the mean value.

Z-score:
The z-score indicates how many standard deviations a result is from the mean.

ABOUT THE AUTHOR

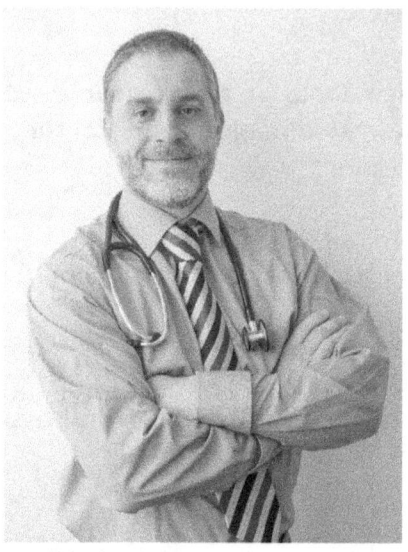

Dr. Marc Barton qualified from Imperial College School of Medicine in 2001. Since that time he has worked in a variety of different medical specialities. He worked as a GP partner from 2006 until 2008 and more recently as a higher specialist trainee in Emergency Medicine.

He has gained a formidable reputation as an exam candidate and in addition to passing a Bachelor of Science degree and Medical Finals as an undergraduate, he has also passed three postgraduate membership exams and two postgraduate diploma exams. He has an active interest in medical education and a wealth of experience teaching both medical students and doctors.

In his private life he is a devoted husband and father of three children. He is also a lifelong martial artist and regularly teaches Jiu Jitsu in his spare time.